How to Avoid FALLING

A GUIDE FOR ACTIVE AGING AND INDEPENDENCE

How to Avoid FALLING

A GUIDE FOR ACTIVE AGING AND INDEPENDENCE

Eric Fredrikson

FIREFLY BOOKS

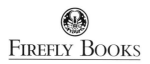

FIREFLY BOOKS

Published by Firefly Books Ltd. 2004

First printing

Publisher Cataloging-in-Publication Data (U.S.)

Fredrikson, Eric.
    How to avoid falling : a guide for active aging and independence / Eric Fredrikson.—1st ed.
[128] p. : cm.
Includes bibliographical references and index.
Summary: Guide for seniors covering the risk factors of falling, general practices for healthy living, fall-proofing the home, how to respond to hazardous situations, how to safely get up after a fall and how to choose canes and walkers. Fitness and balance exercises are included.
ISBN 1-55407-019-8
ISBN 1-55407-015-5 (pbk.)
1. Falls (Accidents) in old age – Prevention. 2. Accidental Falls – prevention & control – Aged. 3. Equilibrium – Aged. 4. Movement – Aged. 6. Safety Management – Aged.
 I. Title.
617.1/0084/6 21   RC952.5.F74 2004

Library and Archives Canada Cataloguing in Publication

Fredrikson, Eric
    How to avoid falling : a guide for active aging and independence / Eric Fredrikson.

Includes bibliographical references and index.
ISBN 1-55407-019-8 (bound).– ISBN 1-55407-015-5 (pbk.)

    1. Falls (Accidents) in old age–Prevention. I. Title.

RC952.5.F73 2004   613.6'084'6   C2004-903116-3

Published in the United States in 2004 by .
Firefly Books (U.S.) Inc.
P.O. Box 1338, Ellicott Station
Buffalo, New York 14205

Published in Canada in 2004 by
Firefly Books Ltd.
66 Leek Crescent
Richmond Hill, Ontario L4B 1H1

Cover and interior design by Christine Gilham

Printed in Canada by Friesens, Altona, Manitoba

The Publisher acknowledges the financial support of the Government of Canada through the Book Publishing Industry Development Program for its publishing activities.

Acknowledgements

I want to thank Greg Webster and Allison Locker of the Canadian Institute for Health Information for their interest and support in the development of the book. Wendy Martinek did yeoman service in the many re-typings of the drafts of the book and I appreciate her efforts.

To my daughters and son and friends who encouraged me to continue the early writing and research activity: very many thanks, and please inspire me to write a sequel.

- Eric Fredrikson

Table of Contents

Preface

I personally learned about unintentional falling the hard way. One day, when I was in a rush, I slipped on some ice at the top of the cement stairs that led down to my condo's parking garage. I landed on my left side and broke a rib. I was 68 years old when this happened. I am sure my injuries would have been far more severe had I not been in good physical condition.

I have been regularly walking and exercising since I was in my mid-40s. When I slipped that day, I was able to break the force of the fall by hanging on to the handrail, and I kept my head up so it didn't hit a step. Nevertheless, my beautiful 180-degree maneuver taught me two things: First, the old saying that it only hurts when you laugh is true; and second, don't rush when you are going up or down stairs, especially if they are made of cement.

During the last five years I have given accident-avoidance courses and presentations on achieving good health through regular, appropriate exercise and I have been involved in various programs and organizations concerned with successful aging strategies. I participated in the Sunnybrook Medical Centre's Balance Program (associated with the Osteoporosis Society of Canada and the Asthma Society of Canada), and have given an accident-avoidance course for the Home Safe Home program.

I have presented my "Stay Fit, Fun and Flexible Let's Not Fall" program at many malls, seniors' residences and other venues. Well-known companies, including The Bay, Zellers, Shoppers Drug Mart, Sears, Canadian Tire and Oxford Shopping Centres, have used my presentations and handbooks in their marketing and promotional campaigns.

I am pleased to say that my programs have been very well received by seniors and the media. I have been featured in a *Toronto Star* article and appeared on City-TV's *Breakfast Television*, as well as on CTV and CBC.

I have already written two handbooks. One of them, *Use It or Lose It*, is about the value of regular, appropriate physical activity for ongoing health. The other handbook, *It's No Fun Falling*, is on how to avoid unintentional falls. In writing this second book, I knew that a very important part of it would need to be devoted to the basics of fall prevention. However, I also knew from experience that the personal injuries and possible loss of independence caused by an unintentional fall really called for a more complete book that could delve further into related subjects.

This book has been divided into four sections. In *Part I: Health*, you will be guided through the process of taking stock of your current level of health – your physical abilities, diet, ongoing medical concerns and any medications you are taking. You will learn about the risk factors for falling, and how to alleviate them.

Part II: Active Living, emphasizes the importance of exercise. You will be introduced to one of the simplest and least expensive physical activities around – walking. This section also includes clearly illustrated fitness and balance exercises that will improve your health and sense of well-being.

In *Part III: How to Avoid Falling*, you will learn how falls can be prevented. The emphasis here is on techniques that will reduce the likelihood of a fall, such as fall-proofing your home and being aware of the best ways to respond to risky situations where a fall is possible. As an unintentional fall is not completely unavoidable, however, this section also describes techniques that will minimize injury during a fall.

Finally, *Part IV: After a Fall*, covers immediate responses, like how to safely get up again if you've fallen, as well as issues like fear of falling and regaining confidence. It also offers advice on how to choose assistive devices, such as canes and walkers, and how to modify your home during the recovery period.

As you read through this book, I hope you will remember that aging is a natural process that we all undergo. There is no magic pill, operation or exercise that will stop the hands of time. However, aging doesn't necessarily have to result in a loss of independence or reduced enjoyment of life. It is never too late to start making changes for the better.

Introduction

As a population ages, the problem of unintentional falling increases substantially. This is especially true in the developed countries of the world, where as a result of larger aging populations and comfortable, inactive lifestyles, the number of falling accidents have increased tremendously. In the developing world, where a more physical lifestyle is the norm, unintentional falling has not reached the crisis proportions as it has in many developed countries, including the United States and Canada.

Where falls occur

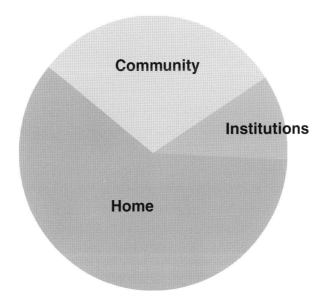

Source: American Academy of Orthopaedic Surgeons, 2000

The facts about falling

Falls are one of the top 10 types of injuries in the world that cause death. In 2000, there were 283,000 fall-related deaths worldwide. Forty percent of these deaths occurred in people aged 70 and over.

In the United States, most falls occur at home, and most fractures result from a fall there. About 60 percent of falls occur at home, 30 percent occur in the community and the remaining 10 percent occur in institutions, such as nursing homes. In Canada, falls are the number-one cause of injuries that require hospitalization, regardless of age.

Contrary to popular belief, falls on the same level, from a standing height, are what cause the most injuries. Common causes of these same-level falls are drug and supplement interactions, tripping hazards, slippery surfaces, unstable furniture and poor lighting.

Falls are the leading cause of fatal and nonfatal injuries to older people in the United States, and each year more than 11 million people over the age of 65 fall: one out of every three senior citizens. Treatment of the injuries and complications associated with these falls costs over $20 billion each year.

Certain groups of people have statistically higher falling rates. These are:

- Older women – especially Caucasian and Asian women
- Users of multiple prescription and over-the-counter drugs
- Seniors unable to stand on one leg for more than five seconds
- Elderly people who live alone.

In Canada, the rate of injuries due to falling is nine times higher for people 65 years and over than for those under 65. Women over 65 are twice as likely to be hospitalized due to fall-related injuries than men of the same age. In total, falls account for 85 percent of all injuries requiring hospitalization for people aged 50 plus.

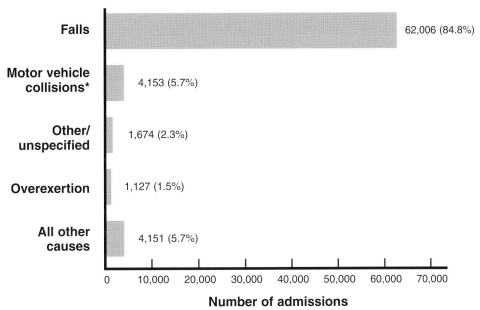

Causes of injury admissions in seniors (>65 years), Canada, 1999/2000

- Falls: 62,006 (84.8%)
- Motor vehicle collisions*: 4,153 (5.7%)
- Other/unspecified: 1,674 (2.3%)
- Overexertion: 1,127 (1.5%)
- All other causes: 4,151 (5.7%)

Number of admissions

*Excludes cycling

Source: National Trauma Registry/CIHI, 2002.

Falling and hip fractures

The most common fall-related injuries are fractures of the hip, spine or forearm. It is estimated that 90 percent of hip fractures are the result of a fall; they are the most serious type of injury and lead to the greatest number of health problems and deaths. In the United States, hospital admissions for hip fractures among people over 65 have steadily increased, from 230,000 admissions in 1988 to 338,000 in 1999. By the year 2040, the number of hospital admissions is expected to exceed 500,000.

Hospital admissions for hip fractures among people age 65+	
Year	**Number of admissions**
1988	230,000
1999	338,000
2040*	500,000
*Estimated Source: U.S. National Center for Disease Control	

Women sustain about 80 percent of all hip fractures. Whether you are male or female, however, hip-fracture rates greatly increase with age. People aged 85 and up are 10 to 15 times more likely to suffer hip fractures than are people aged 60 to 65.

Tragically, nearly one-quarter of all hip-fracture patients die within 12 months of the fracture due to complications related to the injury during the recovery period.

Reducing the risks

Although all this information might seem dismal there is a bright side. By taking direct action to improve your physical condition and balancing abilities, and by learning how to fall-proof your home and move about safely, you can significantly reduce the possibility of a serious fall.

According to one research study, effective fall prevention programs offered to seniors have reduced the incidence of falls by 30 to 50 percent. This is because many of the risk factors that increase the likelihood of a fall can be changed for the better.

Risk factors	Alleviated by
Lower body weakness	Increasing your lower body strength and improving your balance through regular physical activity and strength and balance exercises
Vision changes	Having an eye doctor check your vision at least once a year
Taking four or more medications or supplements daily or any psychoactive medications	Asking your doctor or a pharmacist to review all the medications you take to minimize the likelihood of side-effects and interactions
Environmental factors	Learning how to fall-proof your home and being aware of external conditions that can increase your chance of a fall

PART I

Health

CHAPTER 1

Taking Stock

The first step is to assess your current health, taking into account your physical abilities and disabilities, medical concerns, the medications you are taking and your dietary habits. As mentioned in the introduction, there are a number of risk factors that increase the likelihood of an unintentional fall, including taking four or more medications and some physical ailments. Reviewing all of these factors will put you on the right path to alleviate the risk of a serious fall.

Healthcare

One action we all must take is to have regular medical check-ups by a qualified healthcare provider. It is vital that you have a satisfying relationship with this person, whatever the type of medicine that is practiced. Just because you've been going to the same family physician out of habit for the last 20 years doesn't mean you need to stick with him or her. Good two-way communication is vital.

If you would like to find a new doctor, talk to your friends about theirs. If you have misgivings about the first doctor you meet, try another.

It is a good idea to have a thorough physical examination each year. *All* health concerns should be covered at this time. It is easy to let common aggravations like seasonal allergies or digestion problems fall by the wayside to more serious concerns. If you smoke, you should talk to your healthcare provider about quitting strategies. Smoking is a difficult addiction to overcome – as a former smoker, I know. However, the benefits of quitting can not be overemphasized.

Also be sure to visit your eye doctor regularly. In addition to checking your vision and altering your eyeglass prescription, an optometrist or opthamologist can check for eye conditions such as cataracts and glaucoma.

You may find it useful to make a list of your health concerns, and alongside each concern write any treatments received in the past or those that you are currently undergoing. You may even write in what treatments seemed to help and what didn't. This is especially useful when visiting a doctor you've never seen before.

Date:		
Health concerns	Treatment	Comments

Medications

As we get older, it seems like the family medicine chest becomes a mini-pharmacy – the number of pill bottles can really start to accumulate. It is a good idea to make a list of all drugs, whether prescription or over-the-counter, as well as vitamins and supplements you are taking. This list should be reviewed by your healthcare provider. He or she will know whether there are any possible interactions between your medications and supplements.

Once you arrive at a list of necessary medications, you should ask your doctor if it is possible to reduce any of the dosages. Note: *Dosages should never be altered based on how you feel that day. Stick to the prescribed dosage unless you are told otherwise.*

As vitamins and supplements are now endlessly being pushed at us, it is hard to know what is needed and what isn't. In general, it is impossible to put the nutritional value of nourishing food into a capsule or pill, and my recommendation is to keep it simple: eat good food, concentrating on fresh fruit and vegetables, drink lots of water and take a well-known multivitamin daily.

However, there are supplements that can be useful when treating certain conditions (for example, calcium and Vitamin D for osteoporosis sufferers). Your healthcare provider can make appropriate suggestions.

Date:	
Prescription drugs	Dosage
Nonprescription drugs	Dosage
Vitamins and supplements	Dosage

Physical activity

If you are reading this book, it is doubtful that you are 95, jogging every day and looking forward to another year at the Boston Marathon. Have you shunned physical activity most of your life? Perhaps you were once active, but certain physical ailments have slowed you down.

Take the time to do a quick assessment of your physical activity and note it in a chart. If you don't exercise at all, your comments will be short and to the point! Nevertheless, you can still note how your physical state affects your day-to-day living. Answer questions such as the following:

- Can I go up a flight of stairs without being short of breath?
- Do I suffer any aches or pains from simple activities like getting dressed in the morning or taking out the garbage?
- Are there any daily activities I avoid because of tiredness or pain?

If you do exercise, write down the type of exercise done, how often you exercise and for how long. Do any of your health concerns interfere with exercising? For example, does joint pain or shortness of breath prevent you from taking a walk?

Whatever your level of physical activity, you should show the chart to your healthcare provider. There may be treatments available for conditions that prevent certain types of exercise, or other types of physical routine may be suggested. Also, specific exercises that are useful for certain conditions might be recommended.

Date:		
Type of exercise	Duration	Frequency
Comments:		

Diet

Our diet has a great deal to do with how we feel. Every day there seems to be another study that points out the relationship between the amount and type of food we eat and our health. Whatever the study, the evidence clearly shows that we should increase our intake of vegetables, fruits and whole grains and reduce the amount of sugar and saturated fat we eat, as indicated in the Food Guide Pyramid. Recently information has been presented in many forums about the dangers of trans fats, which are created when fats are subjected to hydrogen gas to stabilize them in a process called hydrogenation. Look at almost any manufactured food – chips, cakes, sauces – and if you read the label you will see the word "hydrogenated." Cut down on these foods. Some companies, at long last, are making changes to produce food without trans fats.

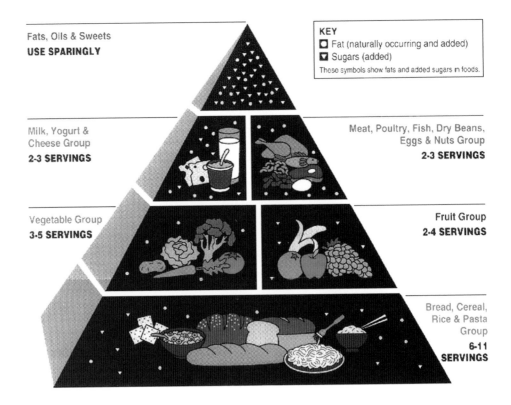

Fats, Oils & Sweets
USE SPARINGLY

KEY
◻ Fat (naturally occurring and added)
◼ Sugars (added)
These symbols show fats and added sugars in foods.

Milk, Yogurt & Cheese Group
2-3 SERVINGS

Meat, Poultry, Fish, Dry Beans, Eggs & Nuts Group
2-3 SERVINGS

Vegetable Group
3-5 SERVINGS

Fruit Group
2-4 SERVINGS

Bread, Cereal, Rice & Pasta Group
6-11 SERVINGS

Another good practice is to substantially increase your water intake. This provides the fluid base the body needs to function effectively, and is essential when you are walking and exercising. It is recommended that you drink six to eight glasses of water a day. While other beverages, such as soft drinks or coffee, may provide you with liquid, they also increase your intake of sugar and, in the case of drinks with extra caffeine (cola, coffee, tea), they dehydrate you. Juices in moderation are good for you, but do note that they add extra calories.

CHAPTER 2

Alleviating the Risks

Although children and young adults fall more often than the elderly, they usually get up with just a bump or a bruise, unlike the older person who often breaks something or suffers a more severe injury. Obviously, the best way to avoid a fall-related injury is to avoid falling! By being aware of the risk factors that increase your chance of a fall or fall-related injury, you will be better equipped to make the necessary changes in your life to prevent them.

Osteoporosis

Osteoporosis is the condition in which bone structure deteriorates because of calcium loss. It usually begins around the age of 40 and women are four times more likely to experience the condition than men. There are no overt signs that a person has osteoporosis. The only sure way to find out is to take a bone-density test. Unfortunately the limited availability of testing equipment means that few people are aware they have osteoporosis.

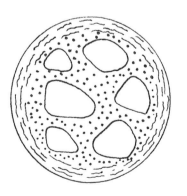 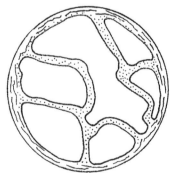

Normal bone structure   Deteriorated bone structure

Because of this, many people, already inactive and sedentary, move around in their day-to-day routines with the likelihood that a minor fall may result in a very serious fracture.

Given that the number-one reason people require immediate hospitalization is injury due to falling, we can understand why the World Health Organization considers osteoporosis to be second only to cardiovascular disease as a health care problem.

The BioSeeker Group estimates (as of 2002) that 28 million Americans are at risk of osteoporosis and by 2015 that number is expected to rise to 41 million. It contributes to the 1.5 million annual fractures at a healthcare cost of $14 billion. Once osteoporosis is diagnosed there are treatments available. But since the majority of the 40-plus population are at risk and will not be tested, other strategies are crucial. The key ones are:

- Learn all you can about osteoporosis.
- Arrange to have a bone density test.
- Begin an appropriate walking, body strengthening and balance exercise program.
- Be optimistic because you can reduce the risk of falling if you take the personal action outlined in this book.

Vision changes

As we get older, normal changes occur that affect our vision. In addition to a general decline in eyesight, you may find that you're more sensitive to glare, find it harder to see things in dim light and that your field of vision isn't as wide as it used to be. Tack on common problems like cataracts and glaucoma, and it is easy to understand how changes in your vision can increase your chances of a fall.

Obviously, if you are very nearsighted, you might not notice that the corner of a rug is turned up – an easy tripping hazard. However, it's not always obstacles in your way that cause a fall. Other common causes are flooring transitions (for example, from carpet to a slippery tile floor) or small changes in the elevation of what appears to be level ground (for example, a patio stone that has been slightly upheaved).

Alleviating the risk of vision changes

- Always be mindful of your surroundings – keep your eyes open and be observant of the surface you are walking on.
- Fall-proof your home (see Chapter 8).
- Visit your eye doctor every year and make any necessary changes to your eyeglass or contact-lens prescription.
- Wear only glasses with your current prescription.
- If you have an eye condition, such as cataracts or glaucoma, have it treated as soon as possible.

Muscle weakness

It is common for people to reduce their activity level as they age. But just because you aren't as young as you used to be, there is no excuse for allowing your body to "go to pot." As I've mentioned, when I fell on the steps at my parking garage, if I hadn't been taking part in a fitness program I would have found it very difficult to hold on to the railing to break my fall. As a result, my injuries would surely have been far more severe than they were.

It is easy to fall into the vicious cycle of inactivity. You don't do as much as you used to because you're feeling tired. But it is because you don't do as much as you used to that you are tired.

Alleviating the risk of weakened muscles

- Participate in regular, appropriate physical activity (see Chapters 4, 5 and 6).
- Before starting any exercise program, be sure to discuss it with your healthcare provider. If you have a chronic medical condition or are unsure how to start, he or she may also have suggestions on the best type of activity for you.

Balance problems

There are a number of reasons why your ability to balance may lessen as you age, including changes in your posture and reduced muscle strength. One major cause is a change in the sensory feedback that your brain is getting from your body. In order to stay upright, we rely on this feedback from all over our bodies, including our muscles, joints, nerve endings, eyes and ears. As we move, the brain takes in the sensory information from the body and processes it, then sends information back. The result is smooth and coordinated motion, as well as good balance.

Obviously, if any of the parts are not working at their best it can affect the balance and coordination of the whole body. And medical conditions that cause lightheadedness and dizziness certainly don't help the problem.

Alleviating the risk of balance problems

- Do the balance exercises recommended in Chapter 6.
- If you are experiencing lightheadedness or dizziness, have it checked out by your healthcare provider.
- If you are taking four or more medications, talk to your doctor about their possible effects on your balance.
- Refrain from drinking more than one serving of alcohol a day.
- Treat any health conditions – problems with your eyes, feet and so on – that could have an effect on the sensory feedback process.

Environmental risks

There are a number of factors in your immediate environment, wherever you are, that increase your chances of falling. These include types of flooring, poorly lit areas, obstacles in your path, deteriorating walkways, as well as many other conditions.

Alleviating environmental risk factors

- Always remain aware of your surroundings.
- Fall-proof your home (see Chapter 8).
- Beware of hazards outside and away from home (see Chapter 9).

PART II

Getting Active

CHAPTER 3

Benefits of Exercise

Exercise is one of the best things we can do for our bodies. It is never too late to start an exercise program – health and fitness guru Jack LaLanne is still going strong at 90 years of age. In fact, not exercising on a regular basis may actually hasten the aging process.

Exercise is beneficial to almost every part of the body. It helps your:

- **Mind** by alleviating stress, anxiety and depression
- **Heart** by strengthening it, which allows it to pump blood more efficiently through the body
- **Lungs** by enabling them to function more effectively
- **Bones** by increasing bone density
- **Muscles** by making them stronger
- **Joints** by keeping them mobile; it also relieves muscle tension, which can add to joint pain
- **Skin** by giving it a more radiant glow.

Exercise also helps you sleep better and, combined with a good diet, can keep weight down – another well-known benefit to the body.

Regular, appropriate physical activity (RAPA)

You can't bring your body back to a good physical condition over a weekend. You have probably met someone in your travels who is aching and groaning after their weekend exertions. It could be a runner, walker, golfer or gardener, and the older they are, the groanier they are. The body cannot reach fit condition in three days. The biggest mistake we make is to rush things. What really works is regular, appropriate physical activity, or RAPA.

If you are very elderly, have not exercised in a long time or have never taken part in an exercise program, are very frail or are recovering from an illness or fall, you should go to your healthcare provider to find out what is appropriate physical activity for you. You may need specific rehabilitation exercises given by a physiotherapist, or hydrotherapy or an aquafit program may be recommended.

Regardless of your current physical condition, everyone should go to their doctor before starting a fitness program.

With the RAPA approach, you will take things very easy at first and gradually increase the amount of activity you do. Remember the key point here: Exercises must be done on a *regular* basis. A good way is to start is to exercise on one day and then rest for two days. Once you feel fitter and more confident, a good basic schedule is to alternate exercise and rest days – exercise Monday, rest Tuesday, exercise Wednesday, and so on. You can then follow this regimen for the rest of your life. Your body will be maintained in a fit condition, allowing you to enjoy an active and productive life and, of course, reduce the likelihood of a fall.

CHAPTER 4

Walking

"My grandmother started walking five miles a day when she was 60. She's 97 now and we don't know where she is."

– Ellen DeGeneres

The best regular, appropriate physical activity (RAPA) I know is walking – gently at first, and then, over time, gradually working up to an invigorating outing. Remember, you should get a clean bill of health from your doctor first. If necessary, you can also get advice on what level of activity you can start at, as well as how and when to step it up.

Stride and posture

The first step is for you to develop a good walking stride – this will become more comfortable with practice. To start, you should first step out as far as you can without straining any part of your leg or body. Your heel should come down first, with the rest of the foot following naturally. To follow through as each step is completed, you should feel your toes flexing into the front of your shoes. In other words, when you walk, your whole foot should be used, from the heel to the toes. Your head should be up, looking straight ahead, with your shoulders back.

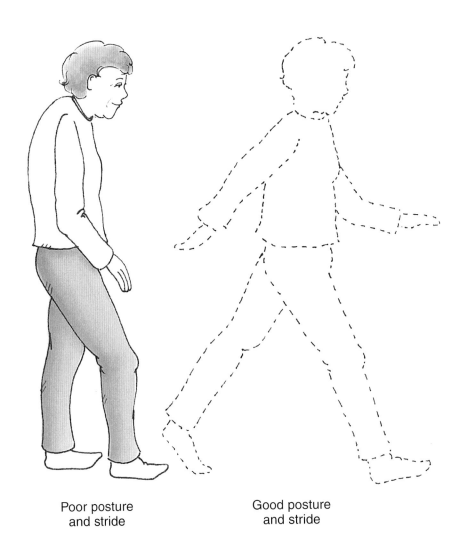

Poor posture
and stride

Good posture
and stride

Warming up

Before heading out for a walk, it is necessary to warm up first to prepare your body and its muscles for the work ahead.

Arm raises

Stand or sit with your feet together or slightly apart, and with your arms at your sides. Lift your arms, slowly breathing in as deeply as possible until your hands meet over your head. Hold the position for a few seconds, then slowly exhale and lower your arms to your sides. Repeat 5 times.

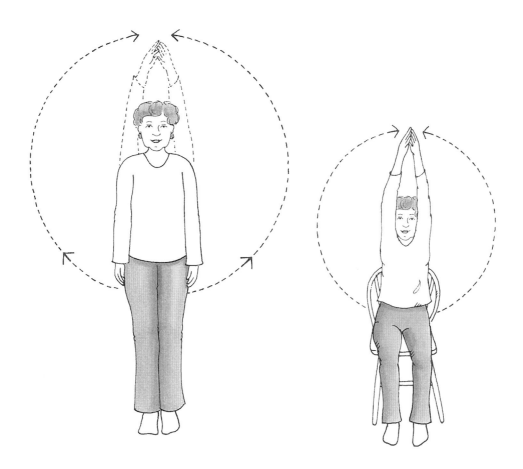

Hand shakes

With arms at your sides, shake your hands back and forth and from side to side for about 10 seconds. You should feel movement in your lower arms. Repeat with your elbows bent and hands up.

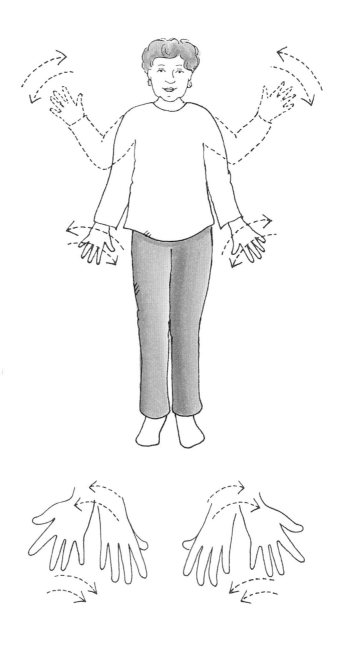

Shoulder shrugs

Raise your left shoulder above chin level, then lower. Do the same for the right shoulder. Then raise and lower both shoulders at the same time. You should rotate your shoulders slightly as you do the shrugs. Repeat 10 times.

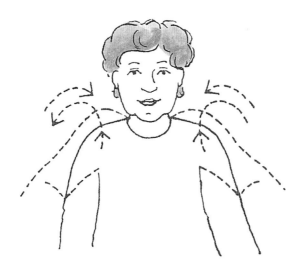

Slow lunges

Standing in a relaxed, stable position, bend your right knee slightly, putting weight on the right foot, and press forward, flexing your ankle as you do so. Repeat with your left foot. Do 10 repetitions for each side.

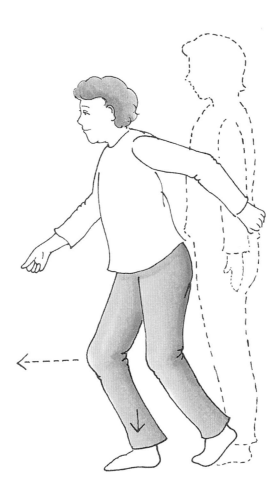

Walking in place

Stand in a relaxed, stable position. Start walking in place by raising each foot off the surface and bending your knees, one after the other. Walk in place for 2 to 3 minutes.

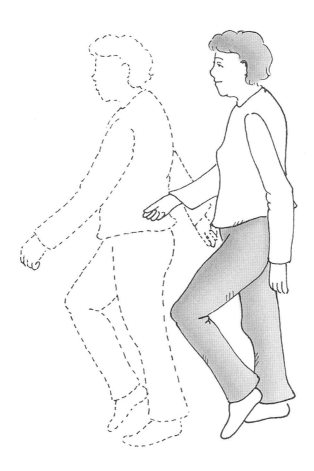

Cooling down

Just as warming up is important before a walk, it is also essential to do a cool-down. The breathing exercise and shoulder shrugs illustrated on pages 37 and 39 also serve as good cool-down exercises. Slow lunges are also recommended. Almost any kind of stretch will also help cool down the body and relax your muscles after a walk.

A walking program

Walking regularly will provide you with real benefits. Walking on a sporadic basis, while very pleasant, will not build up your strength and stamina, nor improve your fitness level.

A good way for you to judge your activity level is to make your first walk a short one, say 15 minutes. If 15 minutes is too much, the walk can be shortened to 5 or 10 minutes – even 1 minute. What is important is that you start with a walk that you can handle, even if it is just across the room once. If you aren't tired out after a 15-minute walk, you may want to double it to 30 minutes.

You should stop walking if you have any of the following symptoms:

- Breathing difficulty
- Nausea
- Joint pain
- Chest pains.

Once you have reached a level where you can comfortably walk every second day for 30 minutes, you can start increasing the length of your walk and speed of walking. Gradually your muscles will respond to this excellent exercise and you will start noticing a difference in your fitness level. Once you reach a stage where you can easily walk for an hour at a good pace, you truly will be getting the conditioning effects of walking and can decide if you're comfortable with that or want to move up to the next level. You may benefit by charting your progress.

Month:				
Date	Warm-up	Walking time	Cooldown	Comments

Where to walk

Personally, I don't like walking around a track. I prefer to head out to the nearest street, park or forest and put one foot out in front of the other, and then repeat. When the weather conditions are less than pleasant, walk indoors at a mall or community center.

When you start out on a walk, it is useful to decide where you want to go. This may sound silly, but I have found that if I have a set destination and route in mind before starting it increases the enjoyment of my walk. It also allows me a good tour of different neighborhoods. Another thing I've done is walk for several miles in one direction, then return home by bus or subway. I find it is worth doing this every once in a while to vary the walking experience.

Walking gear

In addition to being good for you, walking is one of the cheapest "sports" when it comes to buying equipment. All you basically need is a good pair of walking shoes and appropriate clothing for the season.

Your shoes should give your feet room to expand, have good support and, most important, have sufficient cushioning in the sole. This is vital because a great deal of walking is generally done on hard surfaces, like roads and sidewalks, and sufficient cushioning is required to reduce pressure on the internal parts of the feet. If you do not already have a good pair of walking shoes, ensure that when you go shopping for them, you try on shoes at the end of the day. As you may have noticed, feet swell as the day goes on, so trying on a new pair of shoes when your feet are already swollen will allow for a better and more comfortable fit.

You do not need expensive walking clothing unless you crave it or have a nephew who owns a sporting goods store and is counting on your business. Cotton and fleece clothing do the job nicely. In general, socks and underwear should be comfortable, and sunglasses may be needed on bright days, regardless of the season. What to wear will be dictated by the weather conditions. Here is what I've found to be comfortable.

Summer
Light shorts or pants and a light cotton T-shirt or button-up shirt. A hat and sunscreen will protect you from getting burned.

Spring and autumn
Cotton pants, cotton T-shirt or button-up shirt and a windbreaker. Fleece sweatshirts are also a good cover-up.

Winter
Wear an undershirt or T-shirt, long-sleeved shirt, cotton sweater or sweatshirt, covered by a nylon windbreaker; pants with long underwear beneath, and nylon pants over top for wind protection. Finish it up with a pair of gloves, a hat and shoes with a nonslip sole and good treads.

CHAPTER 5

Fitness and Strength Exercises

"Middle age is when a narrow waist and a broad mind begin to change places."

– Glenn Dorenbush

How much exercise do you have to do to achieve definite improvement in your physical condition? I believe that physical activity must be done twice a week minimum in order for there to be a noticeable change in health. As mentioned earlier, regular, appropriate physical activity (RAPA) is the way to go; and the "appropriate" part of RAPA means that you should start gently and then work your way up to a one-hour walking session at least twice a week.

While walking makes for fantastic exercise – and it is one of the best ways to start getting fit – there are a number of exercises that will provide you with increased strength and flexibility that cannot be achieved by walking alone. These exercises are outlined in the remainder of this chapter.

Remember, it's a lot easier to walk or exercise on an empty stomach, so you should schedule your sessions before breakfast, lunch or dinner. You may prefer to walk on one day and do your exercises on another – that's fine. The main thing is that you do the walking and exercise on a regular basis for the rest of your long life.

Warm-ups

1. Stand upright, with stomach and buttocks drawn in, arms at your sides and feet slightly apart. Slowly raise your arms over your head, stretching them out as straight as possible till your palms meet. Slowly bring your extended arms back to your sides. Repeat 5 times.

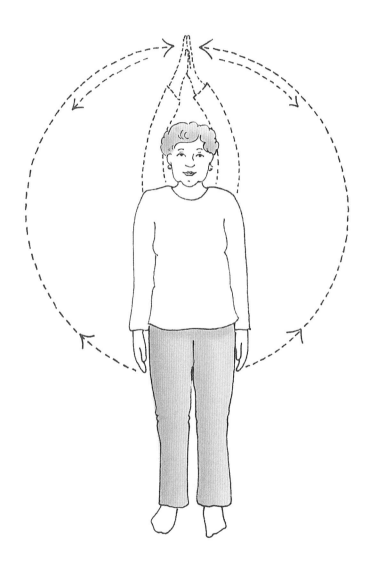

2. Repeat warm-up exercise #1, but have the back of your hands touch over your head. Repeat 5 times.

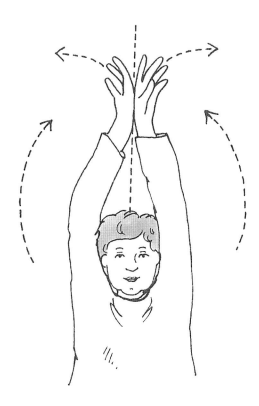

3. Standing comfortably, extend both arms in front of you and rotate them clockwise in a wide arc. You should feel your shoulders and upper body muscles being stretched. If you feel any discomfort, start with a smaller arc and gradually increase the rotation. Circle clockwise in this way 5 times, then repeat 5 times circling counterclockwise.

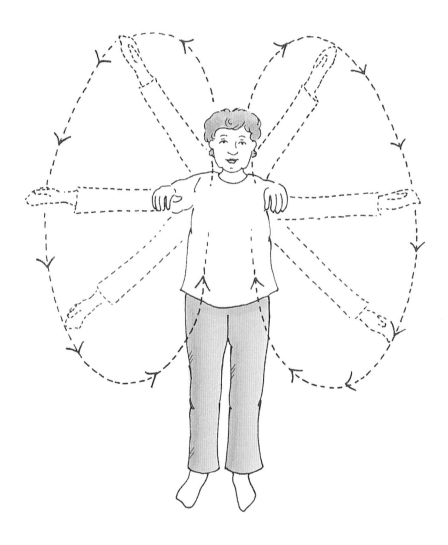

4. Extend your right foot ahead of your left foot. Ensure you are balanced and comfortable. Place your weight on your right foot, bend your right knee, then lift and extend your right and left arms to shoulder height. Bring weight back to both feet and lower arm. Then repeat with the left foot in front. Repeat 5 times with each leg.

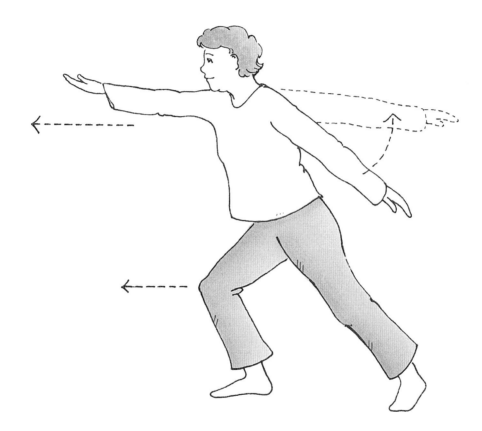

5. Stand upright with stomach and buttocks drawn in, feet hip-width apart and arms extended and parallel to the floor. Rotate the trunk of your body, hips, knees and ankles slowly to the right, as far as you can comfortably manage. Return to center, then repeat to the left. Repeat 5 times.

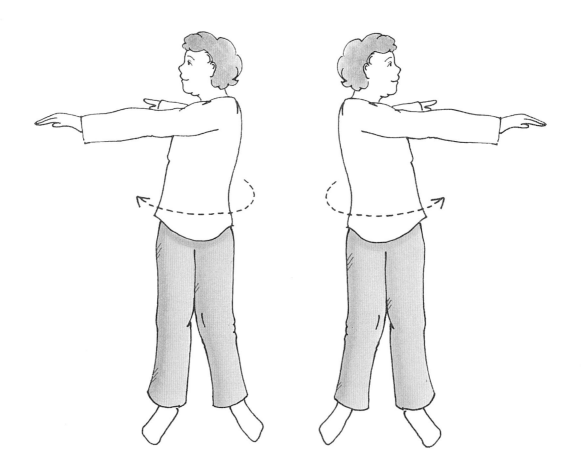

6. Repeat the previous exercise, you may sit in a chair if you wish, but as you rotate your body, also rotate your arms and hands. Change the direction of your arm rotation with each repetition of the exercise. Repeat 5 times. You may also want to include some of the exercises from pages 37–41 as part of your warm-up routine.

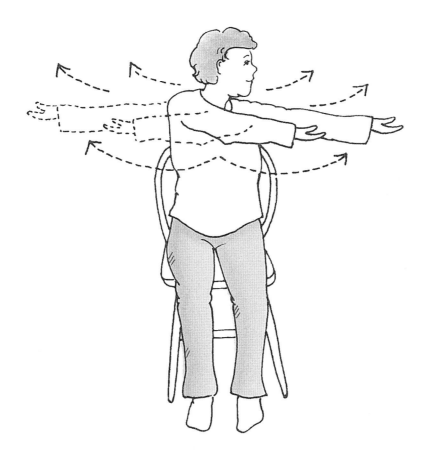

Bending exercises

1. Stand with arms at your sides, with your stomach and buttocks drawn in and your feet comfortably apart. Fully extend your left arm and raise it over your head while bending your torso sideways to the right as far as you comfortably can. Repeat with your right arm extended, bending to the left. Repeat 5 times on both sides.

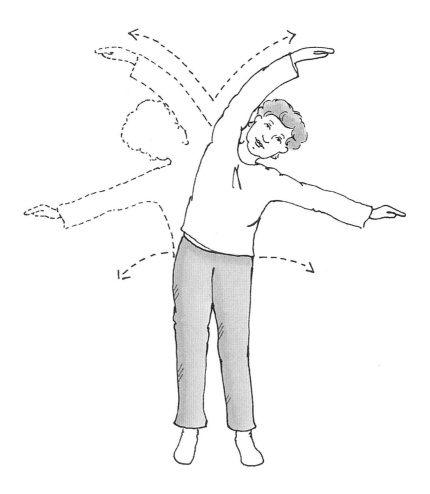

2. While standing, fully extend both arms and raise them past shoulder height. Slowly bring your arms down and cross them, while slightly bending knees. Then slowly reverse, uncrossing your arms while rising up till your arms are up and fully extended. Repeat 5 times.

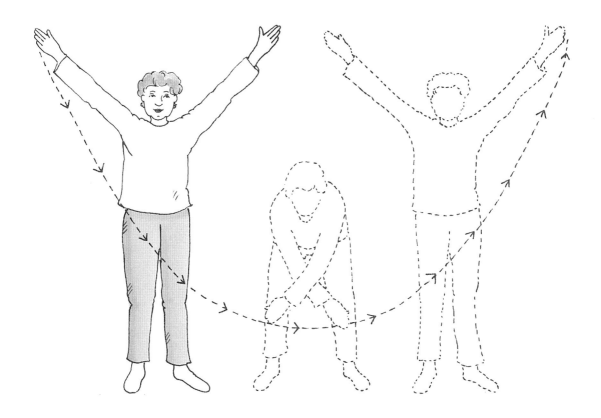

3. Standing with your arms at your sides, slowly bend your knees and lower your body. Keep your back straight, buttocks tucked in and feet flat on the floor. Then slowly straighten your knees and come back to your original standing position. Repeat 5 times.

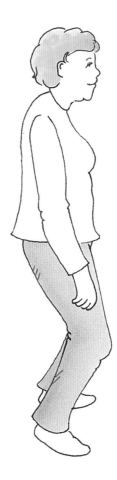

4. Sit in any chair (soft, comfortable chairs make this exercise even more difficult), place each hand on the opposite shoulder and keep your feet flat on the floor. Slowly stand up, then slowly sit down. Repeat 5 times. This is quite a demanding exercise and should only be attempted after you have reached a reasonably fit condition.

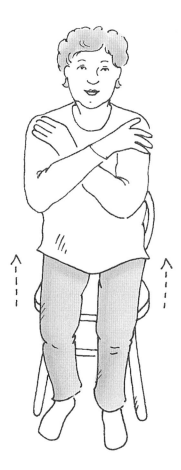

Foot exercises

1. Lie down on the floor. Bring your feet and toes toward your body so your toes point upwards. Hold this position for a count of 5. Then extend feet away from body so toes point out for a count of 5. Repeat 5 times. This exercise can be done seated as well as lying down.

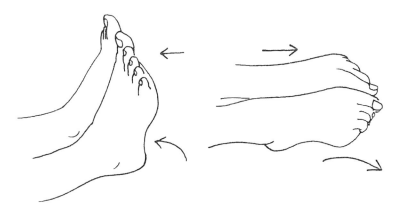

2. While lying down, lift your right foot slightly off the floor or with your heel on the floor, slowly rotate your right ankle and foot in a clockwise direction for a count of 5, then counterclockwise for a count of 5. Repeat with your left foot.

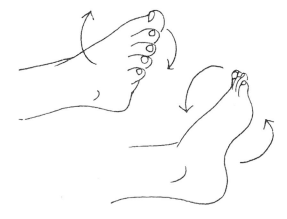

3. While lying down, with your heels comfortably apart, slowly turn your feet out away from each other. Then bring feet together and slowly turn heels out. Return to original position. Repeat 5 times.

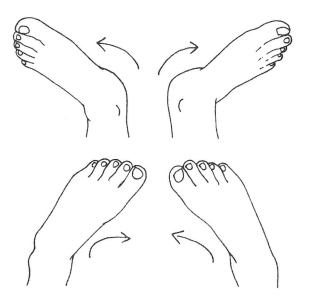

4. Sit or stand with your feet comfortably on the floor about hip-width apart. Slowly raise your left heel, pressing your weight into the ball of your foot and toes. Slowly lower heel to floor. Repeat with your right foot. Repeat with each foot 5 times.

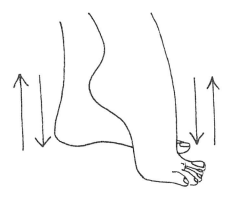

Tension exercises

Many of these types of exercises were popularized by Charles Atlas who, if you remember, turned himself from a puny weakling who people threw sand at to a strapping, muscular exercise icon. His method was in creating pressure and tension by moving one set of muscles against another, or against an immovable object like a wall or a chair.

1. Facing a wall, set your feet comfortably apart and toes about 4–6 inches (10–15 cm) away from the wall. Place your palms and fingers against the wall and press firmly for a count of 10. Repeat, but with your back facing the wall.

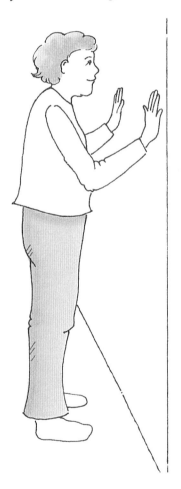

2. Stand or sit with your stomach drawn in. Extend your arms sideways as straight as possible, parallel to the floor. Form fists with each hand, then bend arms at the elbow and bring each fist back to touch your shoulders. You should feel tension in your biceps, triceps and shoulders. Repeat 5 times.

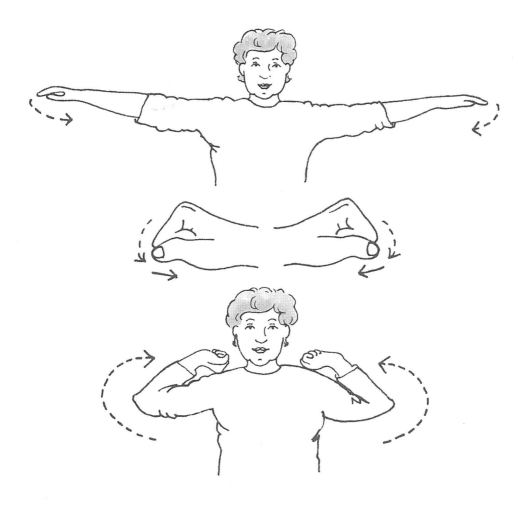

3. Bring your hands together directly in front of you at shoulder level or slightly lower. Press your hands together firmly. You should feel gentle tension and pressure in your arms, shoulders and back. Maintain as much pressure as you can for 10 to 15 seconds, then relax. Repeat.

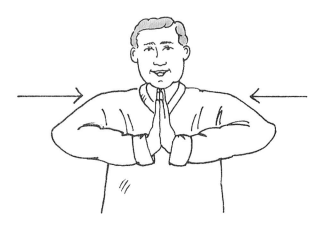

4. While sitting on a sturdy chair, grasp the seat of the chair and pull up. You should feel tension in your arms, with your buttocks pressing firmly into the seat of the chair. Hold for 10 seconds, then relax. Repeat.

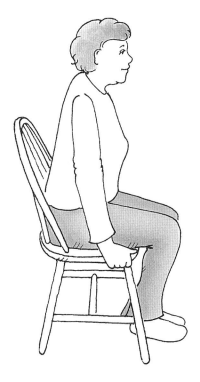

5. While sitting or standing, tense your right leg and strongly push your foot down on the floor until you feel the muscles in your upper legs and calves tense. Hold the position for count of 5. Do the same with your left leg. Repeat with each leg 5 times.

6. Marching in place is an excellent warm-up. Start easily by walking in place for a minute or two. Gradually move your knees higher as you progress. March in place for up to 5 minutes.

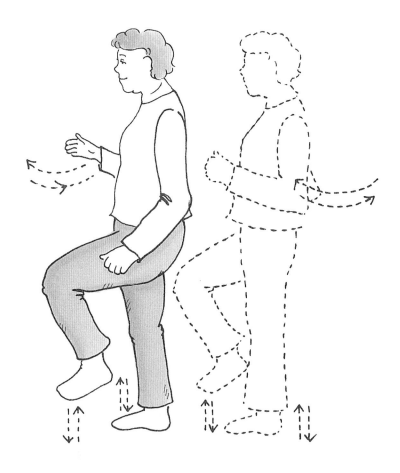

Hand exercises

Although the following exercises aren't strictly for fitness, they are essential for people using computers, typewriters and so on, which require hand and finger use on a regular basis. Not only are they excellent for avoiding repetitive injury problems, but they will also help you retain hand flexibility if you suffer from arthritis.

1. Clench your hands and fingers to form fists, then extend your fingers, as widely spaced as you can, for a count of 5. Relax, then repeat.

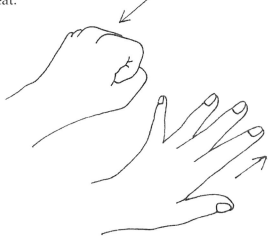

2. Extend and bring each finger one at a time to the tip of your thumb and gently press for a count of 5.

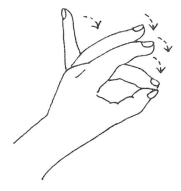

3. Rotate each finger clockwise several times, then counterclockwise.

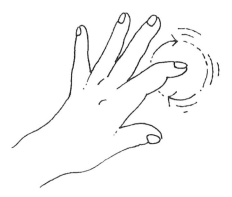

4. Clench hands to form a fist, then raise and lower each finger, one at a time. (Note that your ring finger will not rise as far as the others. This is normal.)

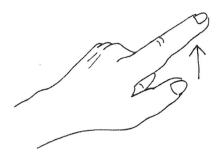

CHAPTER 6

Balance Exercises

"Age is a question of mind over matter. If you don't mind, it doesn't matter."

– Satchel Paige

As we age there is a decline in the body's systems that give us the ability to balance and maintain proper posture. Balance is controlled by the body's ability to take information from the nerve endings in various parts of the body, including muscles, tendons, joints and the inner ear. As we move around, this sensory information is sent to the brain and blended with sight information. The result should be smooth, coordinated motion when moving and good balance when standing.

Knowing this, it is easy to understand how your balancing ability can be severely affected by a variety of medical conditions, including:

- Declining vision
- Inner ear disturbances
- A stroke
- Foot problems and injuries,
- Joint pain
- Arthritis.

Balancing ability is also affected by the natural slowing down of reaction time due to the aging process.

One of the major reasons why older people in supposedly good health lose their balancing ability is a loss of flexibility and muscle strength. Fortunately, this can be helped by doing general physical exercise, including walking on a regular basis, as well as specific balance enhancement exercises that can easily be learned.

Balance exercises are as important as the fitness exercises and walking routines already covered in this book. The same RAPA (regular, appropriate physical activity) rule applies – it is a good idea to do these exercises twice a week minimum. For people of over 50, I recommend a selection of these exercises at least three times a week. If this is too strenuous at first, you should start by doing them once a week, then increase the rate to twice or three times a week when you feel comfortable.

By doing these exercises, you will be improving your balancing abilities and increasing the strength and flexibility of your feet, ankles, knees, thighs and lower body muscles.

It's a good idea to do these balance exercises with a friend present. If you do them alone, stand near a wall so you can steady yourself if necessary.

Regardless of your current physical condition, everyone should go to their doctor before starting a fitness program.

Exercises

One-leg balancing

Hold on to a sturdy support with your right hand and bend your left leg back, standing only on your right leg. Bend your right knee and slowly lower yourself, then return to an upright position. Repeat, bending your left leg. Repeat with both legs 5 times.Variation: Repeat exercise but don't hold on to anything for support, when you have reached a more fit condition.

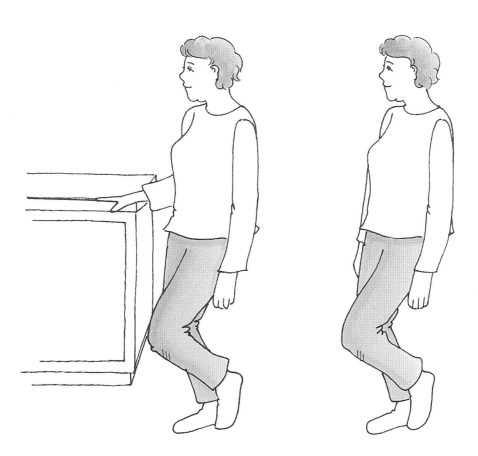

Heel to toe

Stand comfortably with stomach and buttocks drawn in. Walk heel to toe in a straight line for 10–20 steps. Then reverse and walk backwards toe to heel along the same line.

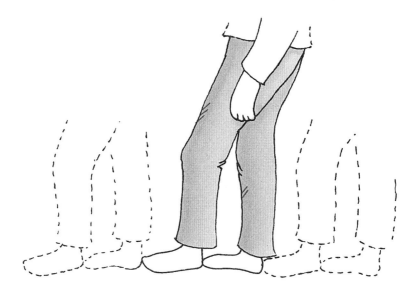

Perfect poise

Repeat the one-leg balance and heel-to-toe exercises, but with a paper plate on your head. Keep your body upright and do your best to keep the plate on your head.

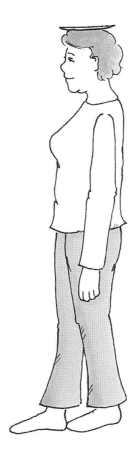

Leg lifts

Stand on your right leg. Slowly move your left leg up and out to highest point you can comfortably reach, then lower your leg back to the starting point. Repeat while standing on your left leg.

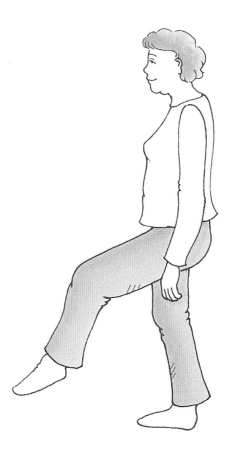

Leg circles

While standing on your right leg, move your left leg up and out to the side. Rotate your leg clockwise for a few rotations. Then rotate your leg counterclockwise. Repeat while standing on your left leg.

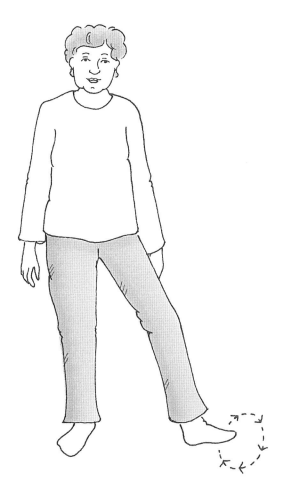

Clock tap

While standing on your right leg use the toes of your left foot to tap out each hour position, as far around as you can go. Repeat with your other leg. Repeat but touch each hour position with your heel.

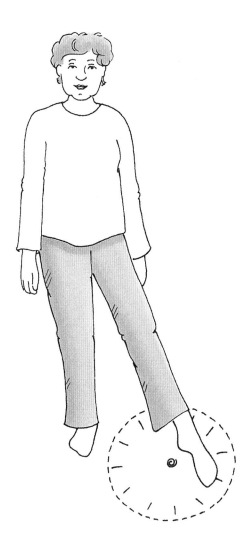

Ball toss

While standing only on your right leg, toss a small rubber ball several times from one hand to the other. Repeat while standing on your left leg.

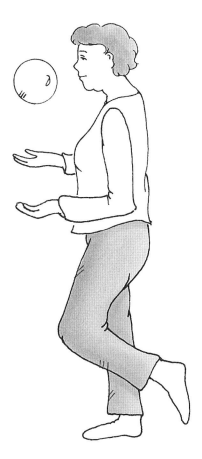

PART III

How to Avoid Falling

CHAPTER 7

Prevention and Protection

Although children and young adults fall more often than the elderly, they usually get up with just a bump or a bruise, unlike the older person who more often breaks something and suffers a severe injury.

The majority of falls by the elderly are the result of slips, trips or a momentary loss of balance. A much smaller number occur because of fainting, seizures or other effects of illness. Most falls occur during routine activities at home or, if outside, on a previously traveled path or sidewalk that may have been raised or lowered as little as one-eighth of an inch.

Some of the most common injuries are fractures, which can involve every part of the body – although the most common sites for broken bones are the wrist, arm, shoulder and hip. Sprains are another common injury. Most are caused by the foot rolling inward; this stretches or tears the ligaments and tendons. Ankle and knee sprains can lead to instability and re-injury if not carefully looked after.

Prevention and protection techniques

My fall down the cement steps of my condo – caused by my rushing and inattention to the weather conditions – taught me a painful lesson. You may suffer a fall by accident, misadventure or just plain bad luck, but you should know some techniques to protect yourself from serious injury.

We can learn a lot from studying judo and wrestling. An integral part of these sports involve falling on or being thrown to a surface, and the participants are *taught* how to protect themselves during the fall. Efforts are made to protect the vulnerable parts of the body from injury by absorbing the impact and shock – done by positioning the body in a way that takes up the impact over a larger and less vulnerable body area. The basic idea is to protect the key areas of the body like the spine, head and hip from injury by sacrificing the less crucial areas.

In other sports, like cycling or in-line skating, where falling can potentially cause a serious injury, protective padding and helmets are worn. During an everyday, unintentional fall we're usually not wearing protective padding, so developing a safe falling technique makes good sense.

The following is an illustrated section on some of the more common falling situations. For each type of situation, there are preventative techniques you can use to avoid falling, as well as protective techniques to use if you do fall. These techniques strive to protect your spine, head and hips as a first priority and to sacrifice other parts of the body that are not as crucial and can be more easily restored. Any fall will be painful, of course, but if you are able to avoid major fractures and severe head impacts, your chances of resuming a normal and independent life are much better.

Same-level falls

Although it may be surprising, this is where the majority of falls take place. These falls often occur in familiar areas such as a hallway from a bedroom to a bathroom or on a stretch of pavement or sidewalk that the person has walked on many times before. I once read about an elderly woman who used to regularly walk across a concrete patio. On the day of her fall, however, heavy rains made one of the concrete patio paving stones heave slightly, by just one-eighth of an inch. She didn't notice this change and caught the toe of her shoe on the protruding stone. She tripped, lost her balance, and fell on her right side, breaking her elbow and hip.

Other common causes of same-level falls are slippery surfaces and tripping over objects.

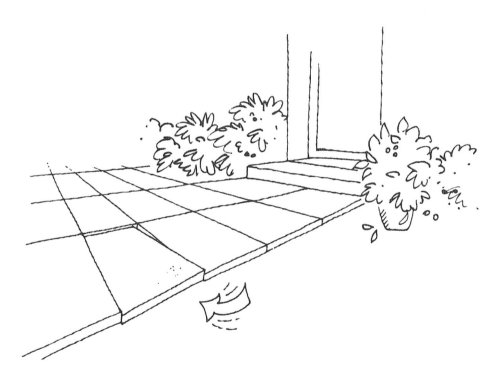

Prevention and protection

To prevent same-level falls, keep your eyes open and observe the surface you are walking on, even if you have traveled over it dozens or hundreds of times before. Be aware of slippery surfaces and potential tripping hazards. If you are walking somewhere new or on a problematic surface, walk carefully, with your weight over the balls of your feet and your knees slightly bent.

If you feel yourself falling, bend your knees to the greatest extent possible to lower your center of gravity. If you can, try to break your fall by grabbing a nearby tree, wall or post. If the fall is inevitable, always attempt to fall on the front part of your body. Extend your arms and try to break your fall by landing on your hands and arms. Always keep your head up.

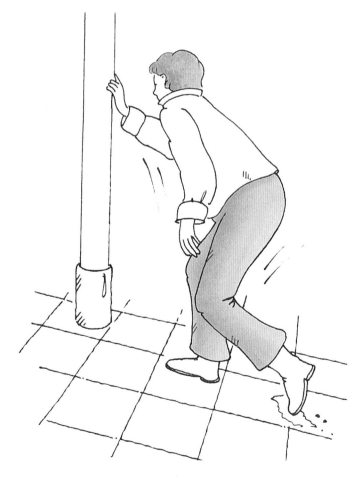

Falls on different levels

Falls on different levels occur less frequently than same-level falls but are usually more severe. They happen when people fall from a higher surface to a lower one, such as from a step-stool to the ground, or when moving from a lower level to a higher one, such as up a ramp or curb.

Prevention and protection

Don't climb up on a ladder or stool if you are prone to dizziness, lightheadedness or are not used to climbing. A fall in any of these circumstances could be severe or fatal. Always have someone holding a ladder when you are climbing it or on it. Ensure ladders and stools are always placed on solid, level surfaces and that the rungs on ladders are nonskid.

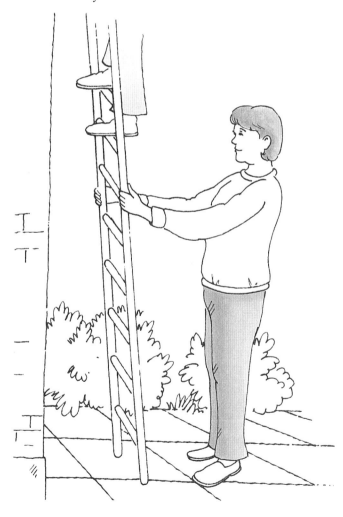

Also, never reach too far to either side when on a ladder or stool.

If you want to move a heavy object from one level to another, ensure you have assistance.

Finally, keep an eye out for broken edges on curbs and step carefully.

If you feel yourself falling, grab onto anything sturdy that can break your fall. If a fall is inevitable, try to land on the front part of your body and keep your head up. If possible, aim to land on a soft surface.

Falls on stairs

These falls are often a result of poor or improper lighting in stair-wells, faulty or loose handrails, slippery steps or carrying heavy or bulky objects by oneself. I know about this kind of fall from personal experience – and I have the x-rays to prove it. Fortunately, there is much you can do to prevent these types of falls.

Prevention and protection

To avoid falling, don't rush when going up stairs. Test the handrail. Use it if it's sturdy. Avoid carrying heavy objects up the stairs. If you must carry something, make sure you are holding the railing with your strongest arm and the object with the other. If there is no

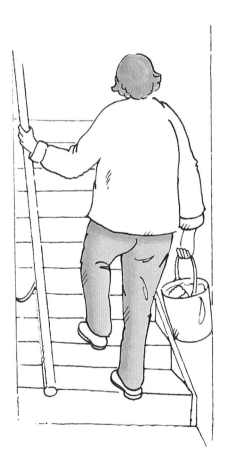

handrail, move next to the nearest wall and carefully place one foot on the next step with your weight over ball of your foot, then bring your second foot up to the same step while pressing your hands against the wall. If stairs are in poor condition, avoid using them. If you can't avoid them, climb them sideways. In extreme cases you may have to sacrifice a bit of dignity by going upstairs on your hands and knees.

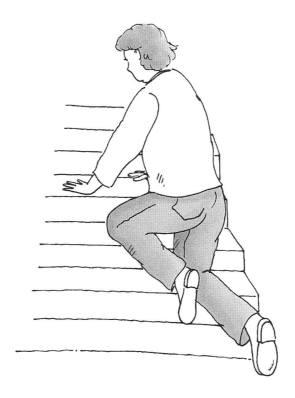

If you feel yourself falling forwards, grab the handrail if there is one and try to break your fall. If there is no handrail, try to reduce your center of gravity by bending your knees, and reaching out in front of you with both hands to break your fall. Keep your head up. If you feel yourself falling backwards, tuck your head into your chest, and try to roll sideways against a wall.

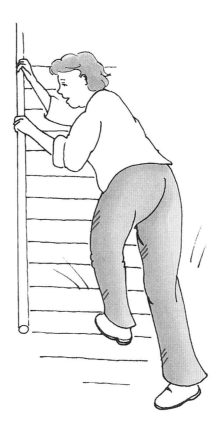

Going downstairs – Prevention and protection

To avoid falls, don't rush when going down stairs. Test the handrail and use it if it's sturdy. If there is no handrail, move to the nearest wall and carefully place one foot on the next step below with your weight over the ball of your foot, then bring your second foot down to the same step while pressing your hands against the wall. Avoid carrying heavy parcels. If you must carry something, make sure you

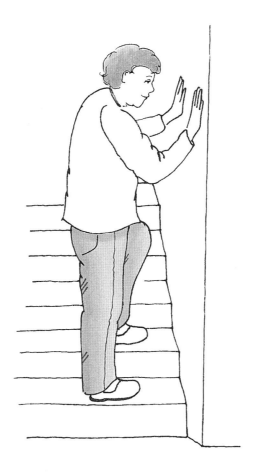

are holding the railing with your strongest arm and the parcel with the other. If the stairs are in poor condition, avoid using them. If you can't avoid them, turn your body sideways to the stairs, bend your knees slightly and move one foot at a time down to the next step. In extreme cases you may have to sacrifice a bit of dignity by going downstairs on your bottom.

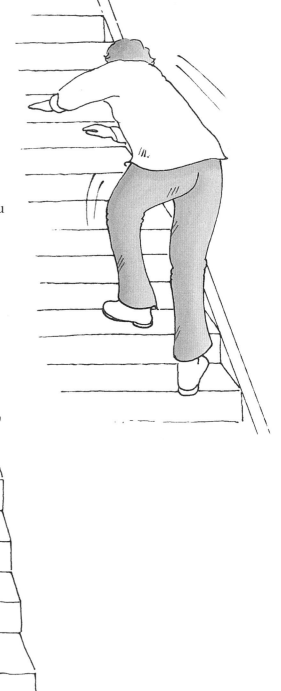

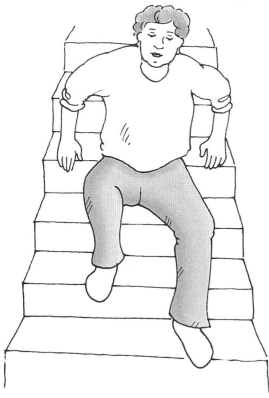

Falling while descending stairs is usually more dangerous than when ascending. If you feel yourself falling, grab the handrail and try to break your fall. If there is no handrail, try to lessen the speed of your fall by pressing your hands and arms against the nearest wall. This may also be enough to break the fall. If this doesn't work and you are still falling, bend your knees as much as possible to lower your center of gravity, put your hands and arms around your head and roll into a ball. This is a technique of last resort, and I sincerely hope you don't have to use it.

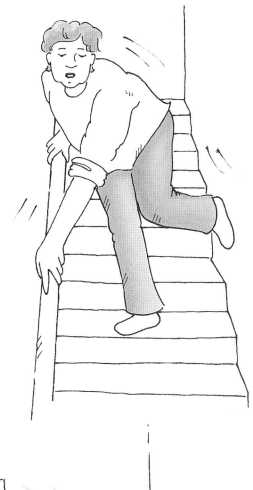

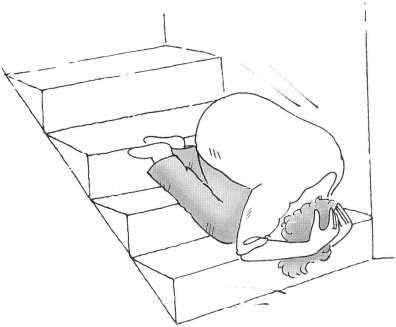

CHAPTER 8

At Home

The majority of falls – about 60 percent – occur at home, often while doing routine activities. One of the best things you can do to reduce the risk is to make some changes to areas of your home, after assessing and changing some of your habits with personal belongings.

Living areas

Keep extension cords, telephone cords and wires away from where you could trip over them. Cords should never cross walkways, but don't put them under rugs, either, as this is a fire hazard. If possible, see if you can have more wall outlets installed to minimize your need for extension cords.

Remove all clutter, including piles of books, newspapers, boxes or other things you could trip over. Clean up any spills and immediately pick up objects that you've dropped. If small children are regular visitors or you have pets in the house, make it a habit to frequently pick up toys they leave on the floor.

Ensure all your furniture is stable. Discard any stools or chairs that don't support your weight and repair wobbly tables or chairs. Also, remove excess furniture, especially any piece that blocks sections of a room or makes it difficult to maneuver through.

If you don't already have one, consider getting a portable phone. If you take it with you from room to room you will avoid rushing for the phone when it rings and have access to help if you should happen to injure yourself.

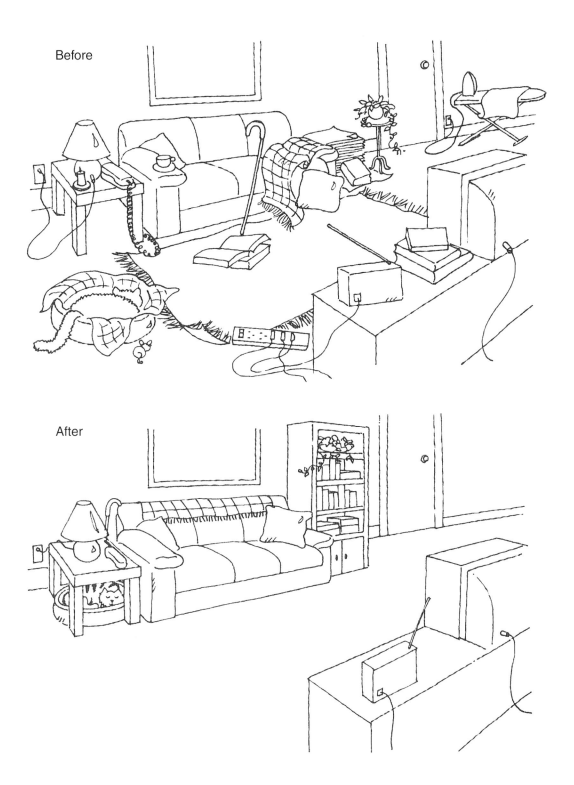

Before

After

Flooring

One of the common causes of same-level falls is a transition in flooring. When entering a room, be mindful of differences in floor levels, as well as thresholds and transition bars between different types of flooring. It may be useful to mark them with reflective tape.

Hardwood floors and smooth tile can be slippery, and high-pile and shag carpeting can be tripped on more easily than other types of flooring. Slip-resistant floor coverings include rough tile and carpet with a short, dense pile. When cleaning smooth floors, avoid using products that will make the floor slippery.

Throw-rugs and loose mats should either be removed or secured to the floor with double-sided tape or a slip-resistant backing.

If you are renovating your floor coverings, try to minimize the number of flooring transitions. Wherever possible, stick to just low-pile carpet or slip-resistant tile rather than changing from wood to carpet to tile, and so on.

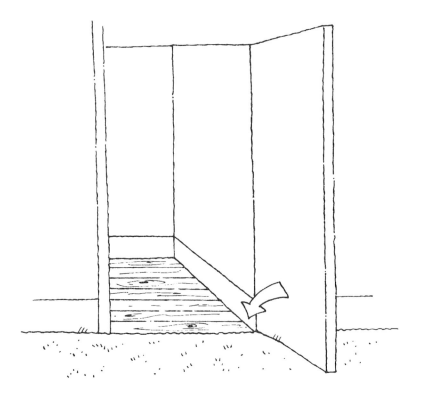

Lighting

Increase the available light in your home. Keep the lights on in rooms you use – don't let an increase in your electricity bill put you at risk for a fall. Use 100-watt bulbs in all rooms. (Ensure the lamp or light fixture can take 100-watt bulbs before using them.)

All rooms should have access to a lamp or light switch near the door, so you don't have to fumble around in the dark to turn the lights on. Relocate lamps as needed, or switch to voice or motion-lighting or you may want to consider installing glow-in-the-dark switches. Also, install night lights in the halls and walkways you regularly use, such as the walkway between your bedroom and bathroom.

Stairs

Stairways should always be well lit. There should be light switches at the bottom and top of stairs. Glow-in-the-dark switches are also useful.

All stairs in your home should be free of clutter. Never leave anything on them. Ideally, there should be no thick carpeting or thick underpad on treads. All carpet or other coverings should be attached securely and slick stair treads should be painted with anti-slip paint.

Staircases should be equipped with securely fastened handrails, ideally on both sides of the stairs. This is vital, especially on basement stairs. Handrails should be small enough and far enough from the wall that you can get a full grip, getting your fingers and thumb right around them. They should also be at a height that is appropriate to you – ideally at the height of your elbow.

When going up or down stairs, always have one hand on the railing. Avoid carrying anything using both hands up or down stairs.

If your eyesight is poor, mark each stair tread with reflective tape or tape that is a contrasting color to the tread. At least mark the first and last steps for a visual guide. Finally, avoid placing throw-rugs at the tops or bottoms of stairs. If they're absolutely necessary, secure them with double-sided tape or a slip-resistant backing.

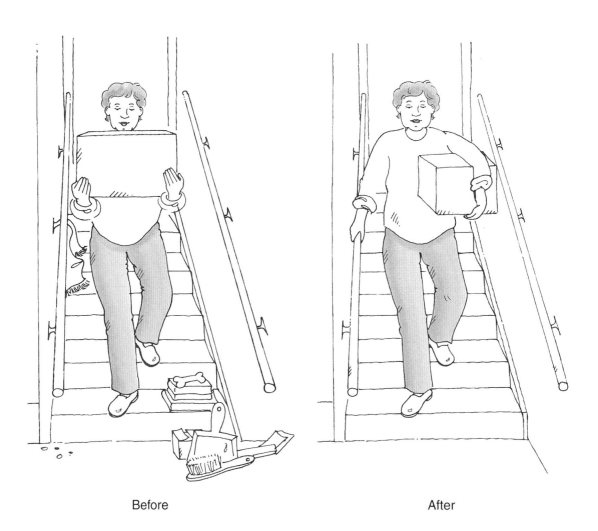

Before   After

Bedroom

As with other living spaces, keep clutter off the bedroom floor. Light switches for the room should be within reach of the door, or install voice- or motion-activated lighting. Keep a lamp, telephone and flashlight next to your bed, and test the flashlight regularly to ensure the battery hasn't run low.

Remove any throw-rugs or secure them with double-sided tape or a slip-resistant backing. If you get up frequently at night, put a nightlight in your room. If necessary, install a grab bar next to the bed.

Bathroom

With the common combination of ceramic tiles and bath water, slipping on a bathroom floor is a relatively common occurrence. So always be careful in the bathroom, especially on wet ceramic floors. Wipe up any wet spots and keep floors tidy and free of clutter. If you have a choice, slip-resistant tile is one of the best flooring options for a bathroom.

If there are throw rugs on the bathroom floor, ensure they're rubber backed and slip-resistant. Secure them in place with double-sided tape as well, if necessary. Line your shower floor and tub bottom with good quality, slip-resistant mats and consider having a plastic chair in the shower. The chair should have a back and slip-resistant feet.

Soap dishes and towel rods are not effective as grab bars. If you attempted to grab one for support, it would probably just break off the wall. Have grab bars installed on bathroom walls beside tubs and toilets, and inside showers. Hire a professional, and ensure the bars are installed at a height that is suitable for you.

Finally, keep a nightlight on in the bathroom for those inevitable nighttime visits.

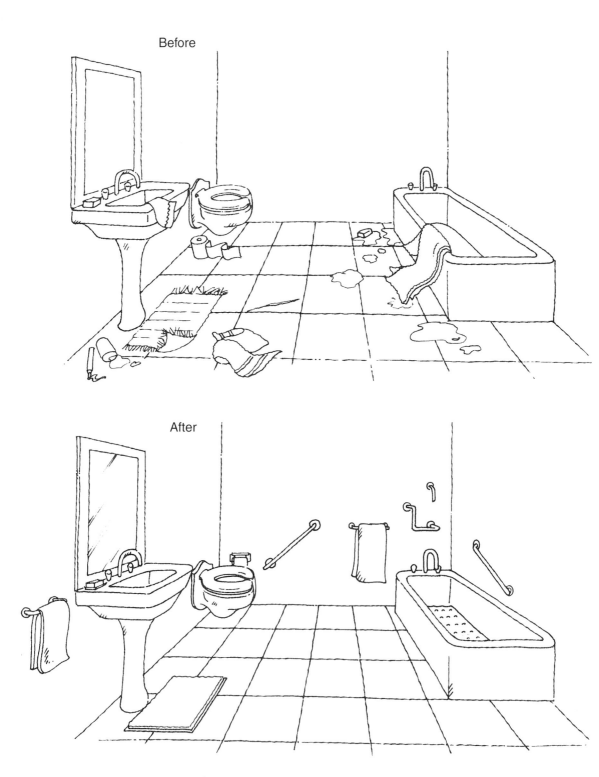

Before

After

Kitchen

Keep your kitchen floors clean and wipe up liquid, grease or food spills immediately. Remove throw-rugs or secure them with double-sided tape or a slip-resistant backing. Avoid letting small children or pets into the kitchen while you are cooking – for their safety and yours.

Heavy kitchen equipment should be on the counter to avoid the necessity of lifting it. Try to arrange all the things you use on a regular basis so that they are easily accessible. Ensure that all electrical appliances and cords are in good repair and rest on a stable surface that is not near the stove.

Before

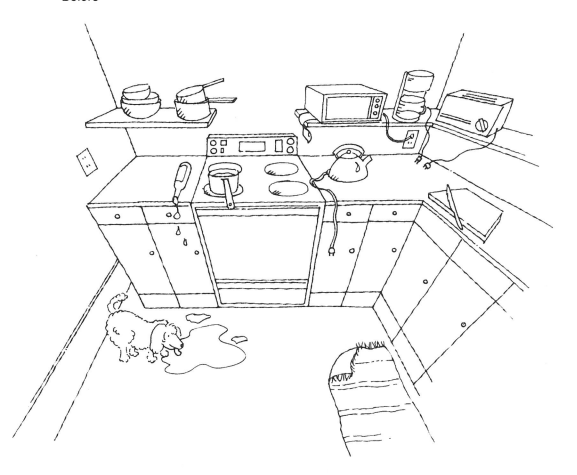

After

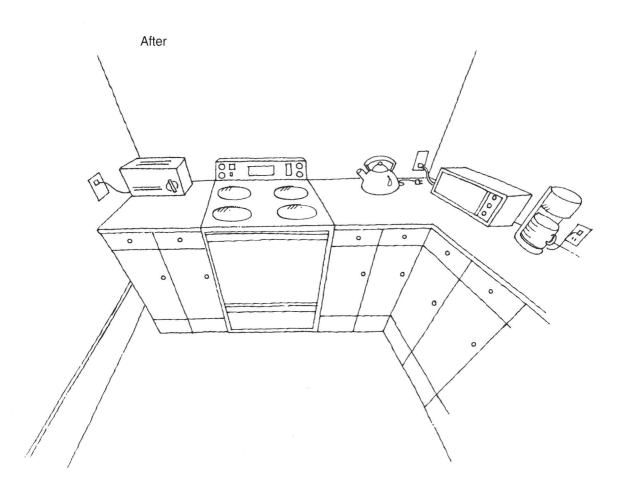

Personal items

The general rule of thumb with personal belongings is to keep them in good repair and replace them when necessary. If you use a walker, cane or other assistive device, ensure the handles have good, firm grips and there are new rubber tips on the ends. Test your assistive device on wet and waxed surfaces to ensure it doesn't slip. A friend of mine recently had a nasty backwards fall when one of her crutches slipped on a wet kitchen floor.

Only keep and wear eyeglasses with your current prescription. Visit your eye doctor regularly and update your lenses when necessary. Misjudging distances and not seeing objects that are tripping hazards are common causes of falls.

Avoid wearing oversized or long clothing. When walking around the house wearing only socks makes it easier to slip or trip, go barefoot or wear slippers. If you do wear slippers, be sure they fit properly. They should not be floppy or backless.

Your shoes should fit. Ensure they have slip-resistant soles and good treads. Avoid high heels and shoes with smooth, slick soles. And as your mother always said, keep your shoelaces tied.

Personal habits

Changing a few common behaviors can also help you to prevent falls. When you get up from a chair or your bed, or move from a crouching to a standing position, always do so slowly to avoid dizziness. Also, drink alcohol in moderation – no more than one or two drinks a day. Avoid alcohol entirely if you have a specific intolerance to it, have never drunk it before or are taking drugs that may react with it.

If you live alone, it is useful to have a daily contact – a friend or relative who you talk to or see every day. If you plan on going out, let them know where you're going. Or you may prefer to contract a monitoring company that can come to your assistance 24 hours a day.

Lifting and moving objects

Carrying boxes and moving heavy objects can be hard on your back, but can also put you at risk for a fall, especially if you need something that's overhead on a shelf. Invest in a sturdy, slip-resistant stepstool with a rail and wide steps. When you need to use it, stand on it firmly. Don't stand on your tiptoes or put the back of the stool up against a cupboard or cabinet. Don't move a heavy object from a high shelf while on the stool. If you have to move an object above your easy reach, ask a friend to help. Also avoid storing things you use regularly on high shelves. For slippery objects, it's a good idea to wear close-fitting rubber gloves that will give you a good grip.

For extremely heavy objects beyond your physical capacity, call someone for help, or get an outside company with the proper equipment to do the job. For heavy objects that are within your physical capacity, always start to lift with your knees bent and back straight. Hold the object as close to your body as possible. Slowly lift up, using your legs, not your back, and carry the object to its destination. Then slowly bend your knees, keeping your back straight and the object close to your body until it's on the floor or surface where you want it. You may want to rent or borrow specialized equipment – like a wheeled dolly or upright moving cart – to make the job easier.

If you are in good shape and plan to move a few things around, it may be a good idea to warm up your muscles first, using some of the stretches and exercises on pages 46–51.

CHAPTER 9

Outside and Away from Home

"Crossing the street in New York keeps old people young – if they make it."

– Andy Rooney

When you're outside or away from home, there are many possible falling hazards. However, they can be handled if you practice defensive walking and keep alert. The main rule to remember – wherever you are – is to keep your eyes open, and be aware and observant of what is happening around you.

Roads, sidewalks and pathways

It seems surprising, but one of the most common falls is caused by tripping over small cracks and depressions in pavement, concrete sidewalks and interlocking bricks, so be particularly careful. Watch for any irregularities in the surface you're walking on. Also, keep your eyes on curbs and don't misjudge their height.

Obviously, you don't want to be hit by a car, bicycle, scooter, skateboarder or in-line skater, so be alert to your surroundings, especially while walking on a sidewalk. Take note of such things as bicycle stands, low-hanging tree branches and uncovered, hard-to-see support wires that can "surprise" you if you're not paying attention.

Be careful when stepping on an object that is covering another surface. I once saw a woman step on an innocent-looking piece of newspaper. However, it had been used to cover an earlier grease spill. Her feet went right out from under her and she hit her head on a pillar. Fortunately, she only suffered a bruise (albeit a severe one) on the side of her head.

Don't try to save time by taking a shortcut across an unusual surface. Whenever possible, find another route. On one of my walks I crossed over a piece of orange construction-fencing material lying on rough concrete. I didn't realize that it was attached to a bent steel post. This put the fencing under tension and made it very springy – so springy that it threw me up in the air about a foot-and-a-half. I landed on all fours and managed to severely bruise my knees, hands and ego.

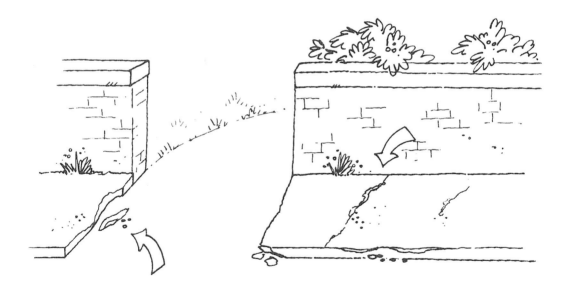

Walking at night in poorly lit, unfamiliar territory can be very hazardous. If it's necessary, go slowly and try to round up a friend. At the very least, use a flashlight.

Do not jay walk. Cross major streets at intersections and at crosswalks, making sure that all cars have stopped, including the one in the inside lane. Also, at busy corners, watch for impatient drivers trying to make a right turn just as you step off the curb. Remember your mom's advice and look both ways before you cross anything.

The paint used to mark crosswalks and traffic lanes can be slippery when wet, so be careful when walking over them. Also be aware of manhole covers, sewer grates and construction-wood surfaces.

Be alert to the traffic flow. Although it doesn't happen often, cars have been known to skid off the road and onto a sidewalk filled with pedestrians. Be especially careful if you're coming into a busy urban area from the countryside. Unlike you, city dwellers have developed a sixth sense to some extent that allows them to dodge things that can cause a fall.

Even if you are a city dweller, avoid the practice of marching bravely and rapidly out into an intersection when the traffic light hasn't gone green. I've stopped doing this since I had a near miss a few years ago.

If you have a dog, you'll be out for walks every day whether you like it or not. So, in addition to all the points already covered about getting around safely outside, you'll need to add another one if you're out walking your dog: Avoid getting your pet's leash caught around your ankles when he or she decides to chase that cute Pekingese. If you own a full-sized St. Bernard, good luck!

Snow and ice

Many of us find winter extremely difficult to handle because it's very easy to slip and fall on ice and snow. Here are some practical steps you can take to reduce the risk of falling.

Whenever possible, stay inside during snow and ice storms. When you do go out, avoid open icy areas. In particular, watch out for ice that looks black or unusual.

Wear shoes with slip-resistant soles. If your footwear is not adequate for the weather conditions, then save them for nicer weather or wear strap-on "spikes" that fit over your shoes. These can be purchased at many drug stores.

If you use an assistive device, like a cane or walker, ensure it performs safely in all conditions, especially on ice and snow. During the winter, you can replace the rubber tip on a cane with a device called an "ice pick." It fits onto the cane end and really digs into ice and snow.

Ensure your driveway, sidewalks and walkways are cleared of snow within 24 hours of a snowfall – for your safety as well as anyone who comes to visit you. Sand or salt icy surfaces wherever necessary. However, don't overdo it when you're shoveling your walk or driveway. If you overdo it you risk becoming faint or dizzy, which could result in a fall.

If you're confronted by ice or snow on stairs, grip the handrail with both hands, turn sideways so you're facing the railing and go up or down the stairs by moving one foot at a time. If there is no handrail, sit down on the bottom or top step and move yourself up or down on your behind, one step at a time. Use your feet on the step below for support and your hands on each side of you to provide additional support. It may look amusing to bystanders but it's better than risking a fall.

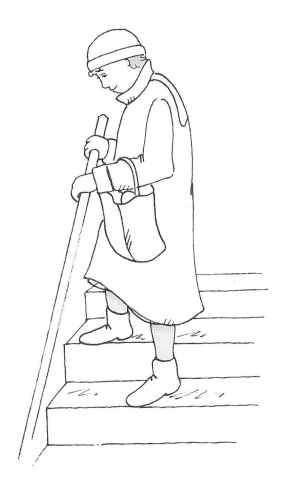

If you have no choice but to cross an icy area, do the "shuffle." Keep both feet flat and pressed to the ice. Shuffle one foot forward in the direction you want to go, then shuffle the other foot in the same direction. Your feet should always stay flat on the surface of the ice, never more than 6 inches (15 cm) apart. If you have a cane with an ice pick, use it to dig into the ice with each shuffle forward.

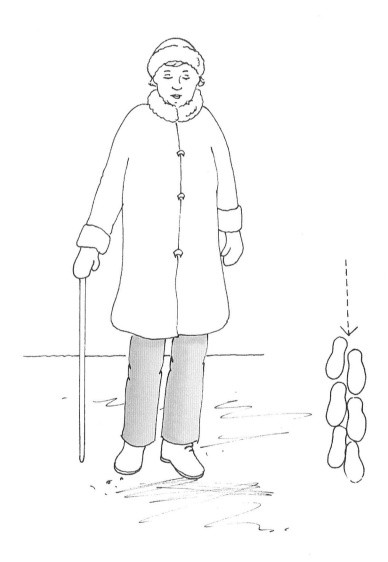

You can also do the "side shuffle." Keep both feet flat and pressed to the ice, but shuffle one foot sideways in the direction you want to go, then shuffle the other foot to meet the first one.

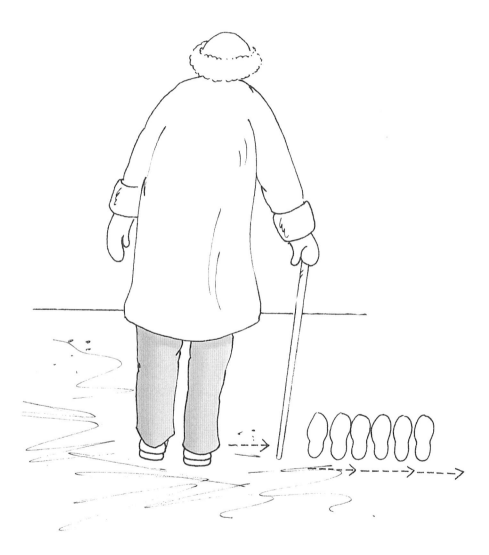

On large, open areas of ice or on slight inclines, you may need to use the undignified but effective method of carefully lowering yourself down to the ground, sitting on the ice and pushing yourself across it. Once you've navigated past the icy area, if there's no one there to help you up, see if you can use a tree or bench as a support. Otherwise, once you reach a less slippery surface, move from your bottom onto your knees. Raise up one knee so it's at a right angle and your foot is flat against the ground, then put both hands on that knee and push yourself up.

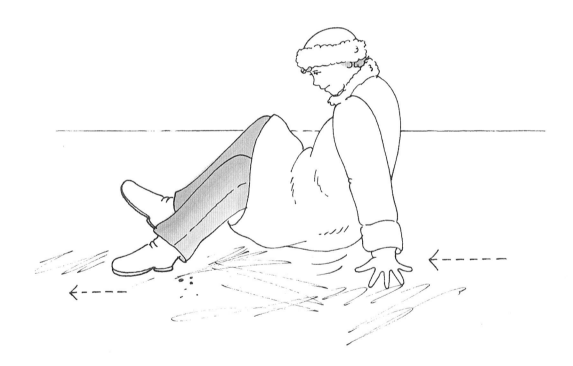

Stairs

The guidelines here are similar to those of staircases in your own home. You may want to review the protection and prevention strategies for stairs on pages 82–87, if you haven't done so already.

Ensure that your outside stairs have securely fastened handrails on both sides of the staircase. The handrails should be small enough – and far enough from the wall supporting them – that you can get a full grip, getting your fingers and thumb right around them.

Stairwells should be well lit at all times, and you should avoid leaving any objects, like newspapers, gardening tools, and so on, lying around. Always have one hand on the railing when going up or down stairs, and avoid carrying anything using both hands when ascending or descending.

Elevators and escalators

Enter or leave an elevator only when the doors are fully open – don't rush the doors. And though it doesn't happen often, do a quick check to ensure that the elevator floor is level with the building floor. If not, take care getting on and off. Move briskly into the elevator and hold the railing. If there is no railing, try to stand in a corner or beside a wall.

On escalators, double-check the direction of the escalator steps. In other words, don't try going up a descending escalator (it seems obvious, but it happens). If you are carrying parcels, hold them close to your side and keep one hand on the handrail.

Step briskly onto the first moving step while gently grasping the moving handrail, and then tighten your grip so you are supported as the escalator goes up. Do not wear loose clothing that could be caught. This type of accident happened right in front of me. The bottom of a women's long skirt got caught in the metal sleeve at the top of an escalator and pulled her down roughly onto her knees.

Moving sidewalks and revolving doors

When stepping onto a moving sidewalk, step on quickly and grasp the railing, being prepared for the small lurch forward. Getting off can be tricky, as you are stepping from a moving surface onto a non-moving one, and your upper body will move forward while your feet will be stationary. The best way to step off is to take a series of small steps with your knees slightly bent until you resume your normal walking gait.

Avoid using revolving doors whenever possible. I've fallen face first into the inside wall of a revolving door because a large chap behind me thought it would be fun to suddenly stop the door from moving. The same guy then suddenly gave the door a hefty push, which sent me into the rear wall where I banged my head.

Some of the newer revolving doors have wide openings and move automatically at a set speed. They may also have a button you can press to make the door move even more slowly. However, watch out for the newest ones that begin moving when triggered by a motion-detector – you may not be prepared for it.

Cars

Be very careful getting in and out of your car, especially in the winter. When getting in, check the surface of the road. If it is slippery, use the "shuffle" method. With your feet firmly planted on the surface, shuffle one foot forward – never lifting it, then shuffle your other foot up to meet it. Open the car door fully, then turn around so your toes are pointing away from car. Carefully shuffle backwards until you can sit down on the seat. Rest one hand on the back of the seat and your other on the dashboard or steering wheel to steady yourself. Then rotate on the seat, lift your feet into the car and close the door.

When getting out of your car, open the door as far as it will go. Swivel in your seat and place both feet on the street surface. Check to see if it's slippery by moving your feet back and forth. Slowly push yourself up, with one hand pushing on the door's armrest and the other hand pushing against the top of the front seat. If it's slippery, shuffle a few steps away from the car before closing the door.

Other moving vehicles

When getting on a plane, pay attention to all walkways. You will want to keep your eyes open for sloping gangways, threshold changes and slight height differences between one surface and another. When moving down the aisle, always keep one hand on or near the back of a seat so you can steady yourself if there's turbulence. If there is a major bump while you're standing, lower your center of gravity by bending your knees.

When traveling in general, your luggage should have wheels and should be easy to pull. Small bags should be carried in a balanced way so they won't pull you over or backwards. Always ask a porter to help you with heavy bags.

On trains, keep your eyes open when you're on the stairs – this is where many falls on occur. Always have one hand on the handrail. Move up and down the aisles with one hand ready to steady yourself against a chair back if the train lurches.

When boarding a streetcar, firmly step up and grab the rail. If you're hesitant when getting on in a crowd, don't be shy to ask someone for help. When getting off the streetcar, be careful of the road surface. Hold on to the rail as long as possible and shuffle away if necessary.

If you're getting in or out of a small, bouncing boat, ask someone to help you. Once you're in, steady yourself by holding onto a seat or railing with both hands and bend your knees slightly so you can move easily with the motion of the boat. Make sure the boat is tightly secured to the dock before you try to get off. Don't step out without having someone on land help you. Again, keep your knees slightly bent.

You won't have the same problem on cruise ships because there are gangplanks with railings you can grasp. Nevertheless, if the gangplank is too steep for your liking, grasp the railing with both hands, turn sideways and move one foot at a time down to the pier. The other thing to watch out for on a big ship is going up and down stairs. If the ship lurches you can easily misstep and fall. So always keep one hand on the handrail when going up or down stairs.

Garden

Gardening is the number-one leisure activity in North America. Unfortunately, there are many opportunities to fall while gardening because you're walking, raking and carrying things, often for the whole day, which can lead to fatigue.

Do some warm-up exercises before you start gardening (see pages 46–51). Crouch and rise slowly so you don't risk becoming lightheaded and lose your balance.

Always place gardening tools somewhere visible where you can find them again. Leaving them on the lawn opens you up to a variety of accidents. You don't want to step on gardening implements, especially rakes.

Don't carry too much at one time, and avoid climbing and descending hills and slopes with both arms full.

Keep an eye open for the edges of your flower beds, as well as sunken patio stones and other uneven surfaces that could cause you to twist your ankle or stumble. If you feel you're going to fall, crouch down as far as you can and fall forward, breaking the fall with your hands. Provided you haven't fallen on a pile of paving stones, you should have a soft landing.

PART IV

After a Fall

CHAPTER 10

Back on Your Feet

I would like to say that if you followed all the advice in this book you would never fall – or never fall again. Somehow, life just doesn't work that way. I know this from experience. When I fell on the steps to my condo's parking garage, I was on my way to teach an accident avoidance class! However, I was in a rush – a prime time for accidents to happen.

If you are participating in regular, appropriate physical activity, including walking and the fitness and balance exercises I've suggested, you have a good chance of avoiding a severe injury caused by an unintentional fall. Nevertheless, you may still hurt more than your ego if you do fall.

Getting up after a fall

One of the best ways to prepare yourself for how to get up after you've fallen is to practice at it. To start, find a comfortable surface and lie down on it. You can recruit someone to stand by and help, if necessary.

1. First, lie still and breathe deeply to make yourself calm. Scan your body from your head down to your toes. Gently move your arms, hands, legs and feet and note any pain. In the case of a real fall, if you felt extreme pain in any body part, you would avoid moving it to prevent any further injury.

2. Roll onto one side. Then, with both hands on the ground, slowly push yourself up on to your hands and knees. Pause for a moment, remaining calm and breathing deeply.

3. Crawl to the nearest sturdy object, such as a solid chair, and put your hands up on the seat.

4. Bend one knee and put your foot flat on the ground, while keeping your other knee on the floor. Then push yourself up and gently twist around to sit in the chair.

You should also practice getting up without having something to grab on to. Repeat steps 1 and 2. Then get on to your knees. Bend one knee and put your foot flat on the ground, then place your hands on your knee and push yourself up until you're standing.

If you are unable to stand up on your own during this practice, it is unlikely you would be able to do so after a real fall. This shouldn't discourage you, however. It just means you need to improve your muscle strength. Go back to Part II and start getting yourself fit. By walking and doing the exercises in Chapters 5 and 6 on a regular basis, you should be able to build up your strength and balance enough to do this practice with ease. You can even measure your progress by retrying the steps every week or two to see if you've improved.

In an actual fall, if you felt pain during any of the steps, it might be best not to try to get up at all. Enlist someone to get help or, if alone at home, crawl to the phone and call for an ambulance.

Regaining confidence

President Roosevelt's famous aphorism, "There is nothing to fear but fear itself," is very relevant when it comes to falling. Unintentional falling is something to be concerned about, but an excessive fear of falling can reduce a person's active lifestyle – which, ironically, increases the chances of a fall as well as the possibility that any future fall will be a serious one that could cause long-lasting injury.

An excessive fear of falling usually results from an earlier fall that caused only minor injury, but created a loss of confidence. This loss of confidence prevents the person from functioning normally from then on. They may withdraw, stay inside and become less and less active in their attempt to lessen the chance of a fall. Soon they're too afraid to do anything.

Unfortunately, by limiting activity, there is an inevitable loss of muscle tone, physical condition and balance, which are the very things a person needs to avoid a fall. The story can become even worse. Other medical conditions can become more severe because of the person's reduced mobility. The overwhelming sense of fear and withdrawal from society may lead to depression – which may lead to *more* medication and perhaps even excessive alcohol use.

Being afraid of falling can also stem from another fear – that of losing independence or being put in a nursing home. Indeed, many elderly people deny or cover up falls they have experienced because they believe it is the first step toward being "put away." Mum falls and the kids may say, "You've got to go somewhere where they will look after you." So many older people fail to mention any small or seemingly inconsequential falling incidents – to their families or their doctors – until they experience "the big one."

It can be very difficult to break the fear cycle, but not impossible. The key element to improve the situation is to maintain and, if possible, improve your overall physical condition. Without this step being taken it becomes very difficult to overcome the fear. But remember that it's never too late to improve your situation, even if you're not very physically fit to start with. There is every reason to be hopeful – at any age and in any condition – that you can improve your physical condition and thereby decrease your risk of falling.

Stories abound about people who have suffered serious fall injuries or have allowed themselves to become very frail through lack of exercise and yet have become energized and active again. One of these stories appeared in the health section of the *New York Times* several years ago.

Alice was a frail, 93-year-old woman who hadn't been out of her bed for four years. She often said, "I'm really just waiting to die." Her niece Bev arrived unannounced one day to check up on her aunt because she hadn't heard from her in a long time. She was appalled at her condition. As Bev had a background in physiotherapy, she decided to try some restorative activities.

Bev began by having her aunt bend her legs for three or four minutes while lying in bed, three or four times a day. After a few weeks of this activity, Bev got her aunt to sit up on the edge of the bed and start moving her legs slowly up and down in a marching motion. She also managed to get Alice to lift small cans of soup with each hand on a regular basis.

After a month or so of this activity, Bev helped her aunt get out of bed and sit in a chair where she would do the arm and leg exercises. She encouraged her aunt to stand and try a small walk across the room to the far wall and back again. This continued for several months until, to Bev's delight, Alice managed to walk unaided down the stairs holding tightly to the railing. After several weeks of watching Alice going up and down stairs unaided, the niece had to go back to her job.

Bev visited again six months later to find Alice a changed woman. She was happier and not talking about dying any more. In fact, she was going to the nearby store to buy food and asked her niece what she wanted.

Was this magic? No, but it seems like it. The fact of the matter is that the human body and brain can regain physical vigor and acuteness through appropriate activity at any age, no matter what their condition. Unfortunately, we don't all have a wonderful niece like Bev, but you can do the things that Alice did to start your voyage to health and vitality.

Remember the RAPA (regular appropriate physical activity) that I talked about earlier? This is the "magic" that can help you restore your body to an improved physical condition; in turn it will stimulate your brain and restore your confidence and desire to live a more active and productive life.

CHAPTER 11

Recovery

The key to recovering after a severe fall is to have patience. Unless a miracle occurs, it is highly unlikely that you will be back to your old self right away. Take the advice of your healthcare provider and heed it. If special rehabilitation by a physiotherapist is required, follow through on the program and do any exercise "homework" that is given. As long as you give it time and do the work required of you, you will see improvement. When you are on the road to recovery, ask your healthcare provider when you can start up your walking, fitness and balancing exercises again.

Assistive devices

Depending on the reasons for your fall and the extent of injuries you suffered, your healthcare provider may suggest you walk with an assistive device. He or she will have a good idea of which type of aid is necessary.

Canes

Canes come in a variety of shapes and there are several different handgrips available. Each style has its own advantages and disadvantages. For example, canes that have four feet offer excellent stability; however, they are often quite cumbersome. When buying a cane, be sure to consider the weight of it – you may want to shop later in the day when you are more tired so you can feel any strain or discomfort. Before choosing, try a variety of canes and narrow down the choices to the one that is most comfortable for you.

Whoever is "fitting" you with the cane should be able to find a length that's good for you. In general, you should stand straight with your arms hanging at your sides and with your shoes on. In this position, the top of the cane's handle should line up with the crease of your wrist.

To use the cane, you should hold it in the hand on the opposite side of your body that is weakened or injured. That is, if your left side is weaker, hold the cane in your right hand. When you walk, the cane and the leg on the weaker side of your body should touch the ground at the same time.

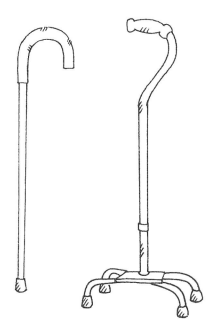

Walkers

As with canes, different types of walkers have their own advantages and disadvantages. Although walkers with wheels are easier to maneuver than the ones you need to lift, they can be cumbersome if you regularly walk on thick carpet or rough ground.

Your healthcare provider or physical therapist can guide you to the right height of walker for you. In general, you should stand straight with your arms hanging at your sides. In this position, the top of the walker should line up with the crease of your wrist. The walker can be higher than this to increase your safety, but as you go higher the walker becomes more difficult to maneuver.

To use the walker, move it about a step ahead of you then step toward it, starting with your weaker or injured leg. Bring your other leg to meet your first, then repeat the process.

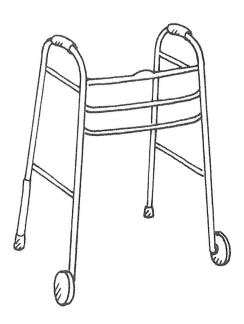

Hip protectors

Hip protectors have been tested in many countries. These are similar to underwear, but they have sewn-in pads on the hips, and also on the tailbone in some styles, which have a shock-absorbing effect. They are comfortable and do offer protection from falls.

However, they are not as popular as would be imagined. Despite the benefits, many women have decided that increasing their hip size by the depth of the pad doesn't cut it. They are useful in many circumstances, however, and you may wish to look into them as an option, especially if you suffer from osteoporosis.

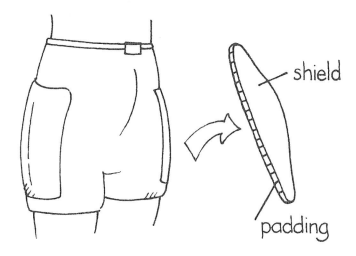

Changes at home

If you have not already reorganized your home so that it is as fall-proof as possible, go back to Chapter 8, review the suggestions and have someone make the necessary changes. The last thing you want is to unintentionally fall while you are recovering from a previous fall!

The following are some specific suggestions of changes you may need to make to your home following a more severe fall. The suggestions focus on places where a fall is more likely.

Bedroom and hall

- You may need to get a special bed that lowers and rises automatically by touching a lever or switch. This will allow you to get in and out of bed more easily and safely. Your doctor or physical therapist will likely have suggestions for where to find these types of beds.
- When getting out of bed, sit on the edge of the bed first and move your arms and legs to stimulate blood circulation before getting up.
- If you are experiencing problems with balance, handrails should be professionally installed by your bed. If necessary, the handrails can continue into and down the hallway.
- Ensure your bedroom and hall are well lit and that the light switch is easily accessible or voice-activated.
- You must have a solid, comfortable chair with a high back that you can easily reach from your bed. Often it is impossible to reach a handrail easily as you get out of bed and reaching the chair is essential. It is also very helpful to keep your clothes folded over the chair so you can dress in the morning while seated on the chair. Many people have suffered serious falls while trying to dress while standing.

Bathroom

- If your bathroom has ceramic tile, have a nonskid rug or mat installed that covers the entire floor.
- Handrails and grab bars should be professionally installed by the toilet, tub and shower. Ensure the height is suitable for you.
- You may require a raised toilet seat. These can be purchased at medical equipment stores.
- Nonskid mats should be placed on the shower floor and tub bottom.
- If you need a chair in the bathroom or shower, ensure it has a nonskid bottom.

Conclusion

At some point in life it happens – you get a wake-up call about your health, career and prospects for the future. Often it arrives between the ages of 40 and 50. In my case it was in my late 40s when I was very busy with business and consulting activities. Looking up suddenly one morning into the bathroom mirror I caught sight of a portly gentleman and wondered why I didn't see or hear him come in. Unfortunately, it proved to be me. As the realization of my portliness sunk in, I remembered that I had a fairly strenuous outing planned the next day to look at some conservation property with two older friends.

That day dawned and I pulled on my splendid walking shoes, thinking that I was ready for any physical test. I arrived to meet my two friends, who incidentally were 8 and 18 years older than me, and we started off on what they called a "ramble." We marched up and down various hills and dales to look at the property. Before long, I was sore, exhausted and annoyed that my friends had barely raised a sweat.

At dinner that night I learned that my friends had been walking on a regular basis for years. They joked with me that I had to "shape up or ship out." I got the message and started a walking program on a regular basis. When I was semi-retired from my busy professional and business life, my walking program continued. I also added some upper-body strength and flexibility exercises to my activity. I think I have come a long way since that day when I looked at my portly self in the bathroom mirror.

Once you begin to improve your physical condition, you will find that you start thinking about what you will do with your newly gained physical and mental energy. You may be quite satisfied to do your usual day-to-day routines without excessive worry about falling.

You may, however, want to go a few steps further and find other ways to keep yourself busy. There are many ways to do this. Despite the concept of retirement, there are many job opportunities available for mature people. There are even several employment agencies that specialize in this field. You can get good information from local employment centers.

Another option is to volunteer for a few days a week. The scope of the volunteer world is huge. Find a cause you're interested in – most of them can't function without volunteers.

Another outlet for your physical and mental energy is to take a course on a subject or program that interests you. A friend of mine, recently retired from a hectic professional job, went into a funk when he realized that he had completed all of the handyman jobs in his house, including repairing the kitchen spice rack – twice. After 20 episodes of *As the World Turns*, as his brain was starting to jellify, he decided to write down all the things he could be interested in on one side of a sheet of paper, and on the other side he wrote all the thing he wouldn't do under any circumstances. One of the items on the "could do" side was "pottery." Now he is a member of a local group that "pots" and he enjoys it tremendously. Whether you're interested in Confucianism, computers or any number of topics, if there is something that you haven't had time for, try it now.

The creative impulse exists in all of us. Often it has been suppressed for years by the demands of everyday living. Now you have the opportunity to write in a journal or even write a book. Your painting, pottery, singing and potential acting skills that have remained buried for many, many years can now emerge and be realized. Don't let the thought, "I can't do this," stop you from trying any one of a hundred creative endeavors. Remember that many artists, writers and artisans did their best work in their mature years.

For a more physical pursuit, you may wish to try some aspect of gardening, one of the most popular recreational activities in the world. Growing things is possible wherever you live, whether it's one pot of herbs on a patio or a large vegetable garden in the backyard.

Whatever task, job, pursuit or hobby you choose, you will bring your unique combination of hard-earned wisdom and skill to it. We've all heard the phrase, "As one door closes another opens." Go through that door to your next opportunity and be happy.

Further Reading

Berkow, Robert. *The Merck Manual of Medical Information, Second Home Edition*. Simon and Schuster: New York, 2004.

Rowe, John Wallis and Robert L. Kahn. *Successful Aging*. Dell: New York, 1999.

Fraser, Ian and Valerie Sayce. *Exercise Beats Arthritis*. Publishers Group West: Berkeley, California, 1998.

Scala, James. *Prescription For Longevity*. Dutton: New York, 1997.

Lutter, Judy Mahle and Lynn Jaffee. *The Bodywise Woman, Second Edition*. Human Kenetics: Champaign, Illinois, 1996.

White, Timothy. *The Wellness Guide to Lifelong Fitness*. University of California Press: Berkeley, California, 1993.

Useful Web Sites

Many local and national health departments and organizations have Web sites that include a section on advice for avoiding falls. Here is a sampling of some of the best.

Administration on Aging
Aging Internet Information Notes
This site provides many links to other Web sites, organized by Consumer Information, Statistics and Prevalence, Prevention, Research and Reference.
http://www.aoa.gov/prof/notes/Docs/Falls_Hip_Fractures.doc

Calgary Health Region
Tips for avoiding falling
http://www.calgaryhealthregion.ca/hlthconn/items/falling.htm

Department of Elder Affairs, State of Florida
Florida Injury Prevention Program for Seniors (FLIPS) is an education and awareness initiative that focuses on preventing injuries from falls, fires and poisonings.
http://www7.myflorida.com/doea/english/flips.html

Health Canada, Division of Aging and Seniors
A handbook on preventing falls for seniors.
http://www.hc-sc.gc.ca/seniors-aines/pubs/Falls_Prevention/Promising_Pathways/promising_toc_e.htm

MetLife and National Alliance for Caregiving
A series of guides on fall prevention.
http://www.metlife.com/WPSAssets/
11908483431050333861V1FFalls and Fall Preventtion 3-03.pdf

National Center for Injury Prevention and Control
A guide for preventing falls among seniors.
http://www.cdc.gov/ncipc/duip/spotlite/falls.htm

Tool Kit to Prevent Senior Falls
Fact sheets, graphs and brochures about falls and fall prevention for older adults.
http://www.cdc.gov/ncipc/pub-res/toolkit/toolkit.htm

National Safety Council
The National Alliance to Prevent Falls As We Age works to prevent falls and fall-related injuries to older adults through outreach and innovative interventions. This site provides links to their report on fall prevention and to articles about avoiding falls in the home.
http://www.nsc.org/fallsalliance.htm

Index